Yoga Chikitsa and Ayurveda: Twins of Wellness

Authors

Yogachariya Jnandev Giri

Yogacharini Anandhi

Yogacharya Dr. Ananda Balayogi Bhavanani

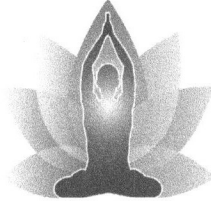

GURUKULA
SANATAN YOGA

Publisher

Design Marque

Yoga Chikitsa and Ayurveda: Twins of Wellness

Authors

Yogachariya Jnandev Giri

Yogacharini Anandhi

Yogacharya Dr. Ananda Balayogi Bhavanani

First Published July 2023
ISBN 978-1-914485-13-8

Printed in Great Britain
by

Design Marque

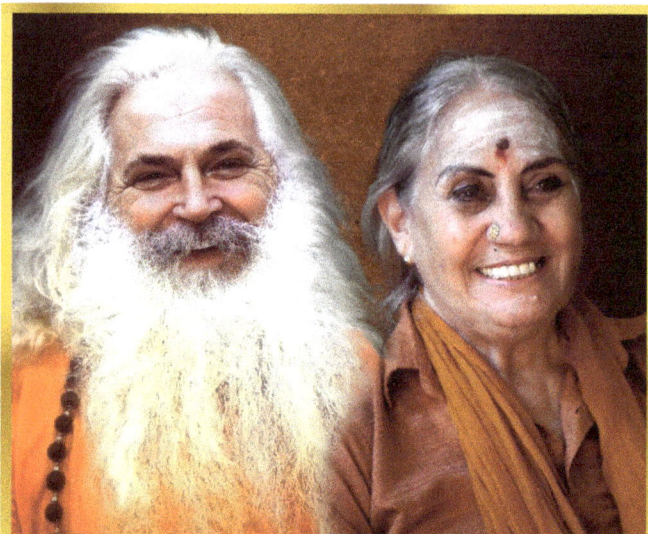

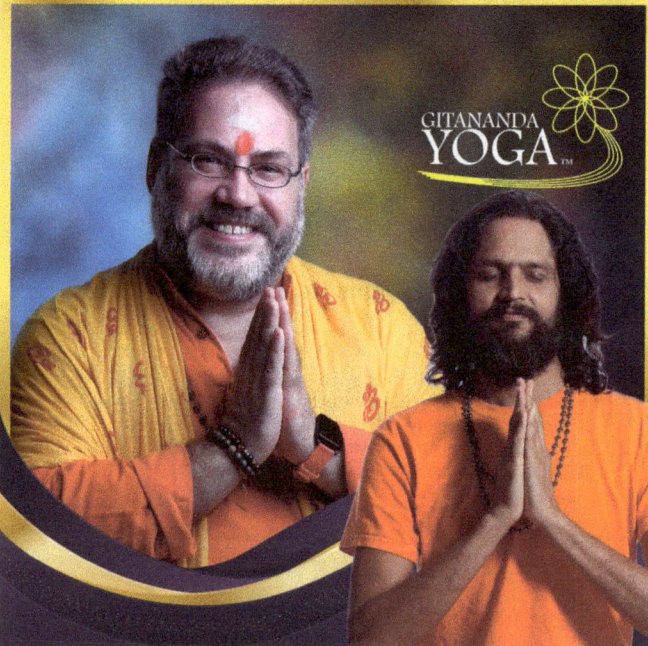

"We dedicate this book to our Divine Gurus Yogamaharishi Dr Swami Gitananda Giri Guru Maharaj and Param Pujya Ammaji, Yogacharini Meenakshi Devi Bhavanani"

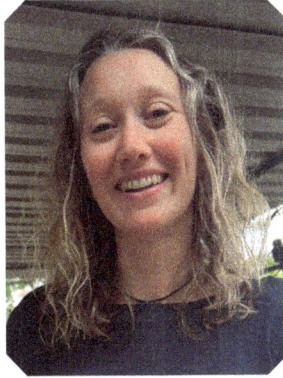

Summary

To achieve yogic integration into all levels of our being, it is essential that a multi-dimensional approach which includes all aspects of yoga is followed. This includes a wholesome, nourishing diet, a healthy environment and lifestyle in addition to the (yoga) practices carried out on our yoga mats. This first part of this book provides an insightful look into the yogic perspective on health, the principles of Yoga Chikitsa and the application of yoga as therapy in order to live a healthy life.

The second part of the book blends yoga theory with Ayurveda to provide an oversight of the role that Ayurveda can play in improving health. Including:

- A detailed look at the three Doshas; Vata, Pitta and Kapha
- Take the quiz and learn how to identify the composition of Doshas within the body
- Factors that aggravate the Doshas causing imbalances and how these can be identified
- The impact of the doshas to the body, mind and emotions
- The benefits of eating an activated diet
- Fasting and Ayurveda
- The importance of good digestive health as per Ayurveda and yogic theory

by Louisa Humphrey
(Senior Sanatan Yoga Teacher)

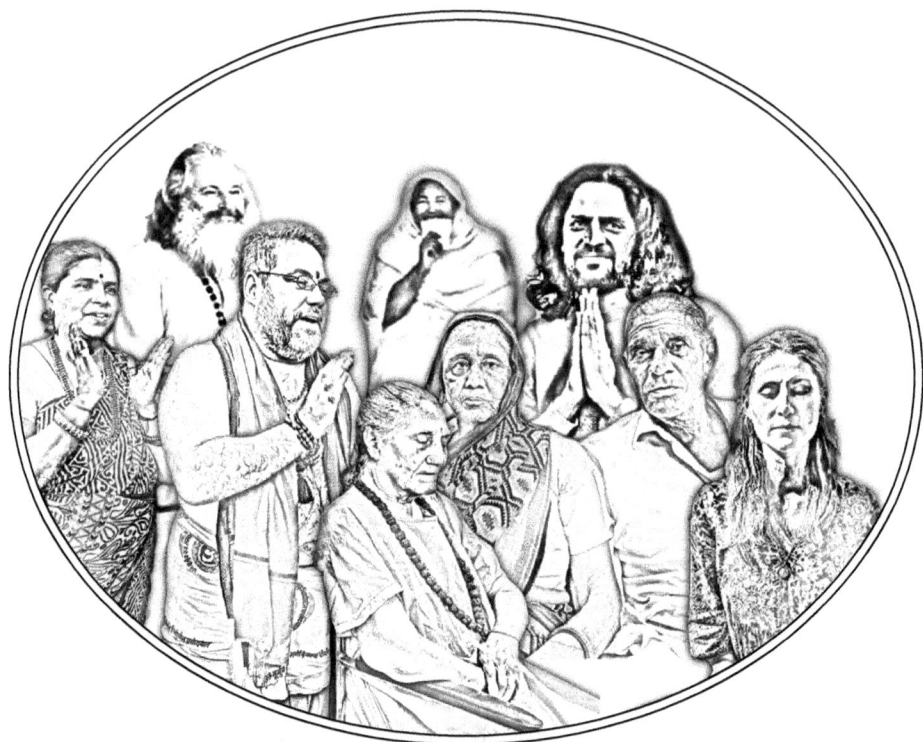

Gratitude by
Yogachariya Jnandev Giri

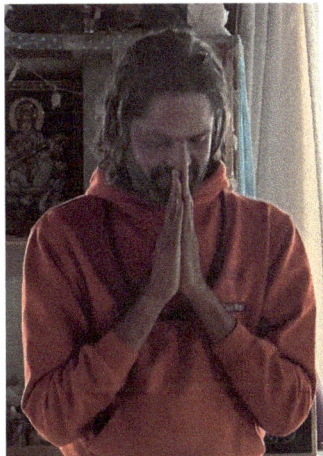

This book on Ayurveda and Yoga Chikitsa is a compilation of research for all the sincere Yoga, Health, Spiritual Seekers and Yoga Chikitsa or Yoga Therapy professionals who wish to use the basic Ayurvedic principles of dosha, dhatus, agnis and an activated diet to support the Yoga Chikitsa Program. Yogachariya Dr Ananda Balayogi Bhavanani mentions that wholistic Yoga Chikitsa is to help the yoga followers or care seekers to attain their full potential. May we all live in harmony with our truest nature. May we attain our full potential. May our diet support our body, mind and life. May we live virtuously and be able to use these truly amazing tools for a healthier body, mind and spirit.

I would like to offer my gratitude and special thanks to my dearest Guru Ammaji Meenakshi Devi Bhavanani, Swamiji. I would also like to offer my sincerest gratitude to Yogachariya Dr Ananda Balayogi Bhavanani and Yogacharini Anandhi for guiding me to compile this book and giving us all their unconditional love, support and blessings to move forward. I also express my deepest gratitude to all the authors and resources we have used as part of this compilation.

I would like to offer my special thanks and gratitude to my three divine boys, Siddha, Mahadev and Krishna, for all their love, support and motivation in my life.

I am very grateful to the Selfless Service (Niskama Seva) of Dharmananda for proofreading this book, and Sarah Ray (Design Marque, Pembrokeshire) for the truly amazing design work as always. I express my gratitude to Louisa Humphrey and Isie Everett for proof reading. Finally, I also offer my thanks to all my Yoga Family and the local Welsh community, all of whom have supported both myself and Gurukula UK on the path of teaching, writing and living a yogic life.

With Love and Blessings
Yogachariya Jnandev Giri
Founder & Director, Gurukula UK, & Portugal

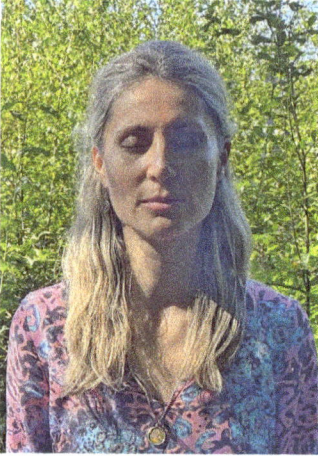

Gratitude by
Anandhi Korina Kointaxaki

This book was written during the two-year yoga therapy training with Yogacharya Jnandev and his team as teachers and students, we experienced that yoga Chikitsa is difficult to be successful without the sister science Ayurveda Chikitsa.

Originally, Chikitsa was referring to both Ayurveda and yoga and these two where not considered separate.

During our involvement with the yoga therapy students, we faced this connection and we thought we can put our experience, our research and our knowledge into a book for our students and anyone interested in yoga and Ayurveda as sister sciences.

I participated in the yoga therapy training not so much as an Ayurvedic counsellor but mostly as a yogic diet practical expert. My love and interest in yogic life made me create a unique system which I called "activated food" because it keeps its prana. In this book we mention the basics of this system which can be practiced by the care seekers to support their therapy.

Yogacharini Anandhi Korina Kointaxaki
https://yogalifewithanandhi.com

Blessings by Ammaji, Yogacharini Meenakshi Devi

One of the unique features of the timeless wellness system of Yoga is that it provides a complete discipline of body, emotions, mind and spirit. Every aspect of the human being is refined by practices which have been proven through generations of the Rishiculture Yoga Parampara.

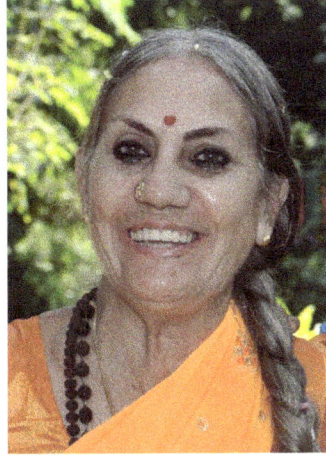

To take responsibility for one's life in an intelligent manner is indeed Yogic. All other societies, including political and religious societies, put the blame onto contrary systems or even onto God, for what is happening to us individually and for humankind as a whole. What also happens is that we become wise enough to accept responsibility for what we are doing now, but want to deny any responsibility for what we have been previously doing. Accepting the Law of Karma doesn't wipe out the past mistakes. It has to be worked out in conscious living. The idea that simply "feeling sorry" or feeling remorse for mistakes, thoughts, words or deeds, sins, lapses, etc which we have done will free using the effects of our deeds is a nonsensical concept devised by immature minds which cannot face the reality of irrevocable Universal Laws. Nothing can "wash away our sins" but we can with conscious effort "work out" the unhappy effects of past foolish action.

Unfortunately, the body, emotions and mind have all been conditioned by previous life styles, attitudes and actions. It may take some time for things to come into balance. Also as we grow older it is more difficult to change body problems that are deeply entrenched. It is easier, however, to change one's emotions and mind as we grow older. That is why maturity gives some semblance of balance of compensation for the past. At least we can look forward to a limited future that is in our control. The past has to be worked out by present action.

- Param Pujya Ammaji, Yogacharini Meenakshi Devi Bhavanani, Ashram Acharya and Director ICYER at Ananda Ashram, Pondicherry, India.

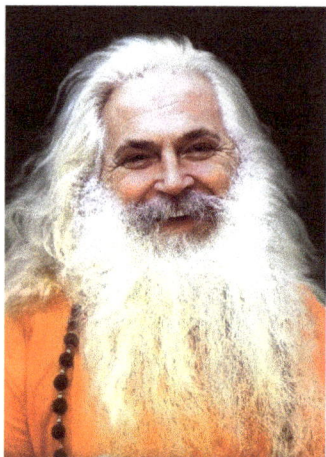

Blessings by Yogamaharishi Dr Swami Gitananda Giri Guru Maharaj

Yoga as a life style has an answer to depression, stress, strain and anxiety. Engaging in the Asanas, Kriyas and Mudras along with the proper Pranayama goes a long way to aid in relieving the condition. Yoga practice is basically isometric, rather than isotonic. Therefore, it has an advantage for all types of depression. Isometric Yoga plays body movement against the breath, while isotonic activity is to be observed in heavy work sports and recreational play. Although the latter does give a false sense of relief from tension, only a personality change can relieve the condition totally. It is to be sadly noted that Western culture has advanced a long way in using relaxation techniques in every form of recreation, sport and medicine, while here in India, little or nothing is known about Hatha Yoga relaxation or Jnana Yoga counselling which are both fields producing dynamic recovery from depression and repression. It is to be hoped that leading Research Centres devote time to this valuable research field. More people are dying daily from conditions caused by anxiety, stress, and tension than by all other diseases put together. Yet, this is hardly recognized in the statistics of death from so-called "natural causes."

- Yogamaharishi Dr Swami Gitananda Giri Guru Maharaj, Founder Ananda Ashram at ICYER, Pondicherry, India.

Blessings by Yogacharya Dr Ananda Balayogi Bhavanani

BE A YOGA CHIKITSAK, A NOBLE YOGA THERAPIST

Yogacharya Dr Ananda Balayogi Bhavanani Ashram Acharya and Director ICYER at Ananda Ashram and ISCM of Sri Balaji Vidyapeeth, Pondicherry, India.

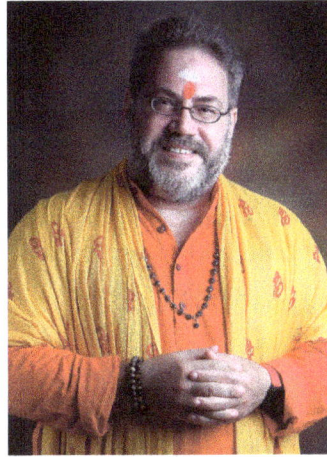

The best ever definition of health may be attributed to the father of surgery, Acharya Sushrut (~600 BC) who defined health as "a dynamic balance of the elements and humors, normal metabolic activity and efficient elimination coupled with a tranquil mind, senses and contented soul" (samadoshah samaagnishch samadhaatu–malakriyah, prasanna atmendriya manah swasth ityabhidheeyate. Sushrut Samhita, Sutrasthanam, 15:41).

Yoga to me is undoubtedly and truly the best means to achieve such a dynamic state of wholistic health.

As Yoga Chikitsa starts to be introduced into mainstream health care, we must not fall into the dangerous trap of claiming that Yoga is a miracle that can cure everything under the sun for that "puts off" the modern medical community more than anything. They then develop a stiff resistance to Yoga instead of becoming more open to this life giving and health restoring science.

As the use of Yoga Chikitsa in medical centers is still in its infancy we must be cautious about the after-effects we may produce by our conscious and unconscious thoughts, words and actions. Better to err on the side of caution than be true to the adage, "fools rush in where angels fear to tread".

We must remember that, it is only when we begin to consciously understand our limitations that we can then grow and evolve multiplying our inherent strengths multifold.

I am not downplaying the potentiality of Yoga for it DOES have a role in virtually each and every condition affecting humankind. As stress is the main causative, precipitating and aggravating factor in every known disorder and disease, Yoga as the potent antidote to stress can for sure improve things for the better.

However, though Yoga can improve the condition of nearly every patient, it doesn't necessarily translate into words such as cure.

Modern medicine doesn't have a cure for most conditions and hence when Yoga therapists use such words, it creates a negative image and consequent reaction that does more harm than good.

We must remember that the wise "know" that they "know nothing", the arrogant and ignorant fools "think" they "know everything".

I would like to reiterate at this point the need of the modern age which is to have an integrated approach towards all forms of therapy. Integrative medicine is the future and we must try to integrate concepts of Yoga in coordination and collaboration with other systems of medicine such as Allopathy, Ayurveda, Siddha, Homeopathy and Naturopathy. Physiotherapy, osteopathy and chiropractic practices may be also used with the Yoga Chikitsa as required.

Lifestyle modification is the keyword and we must not forget that advice on diet and adoption of a healthy natural lifestyle is very important irrespective of the mode of therapy employed for the patient.

I feel that it is apt to end with a Subhashita, one of many witty and epigrammatic verses in Sanskrit literature that taunts those doctors and therapists who do not treat their patients in a proper way and who are more interested in making money, name and fame than in curing them.

vaidyaraaja namastubhyam yamaraaja sahodarah

yamastu harati praanaan vaidyah praanaan dhanaani cha

This may be translated as follows. "Salutations to you O doctor, for you are the brother of Yamaraja, the Lord of death. Whereas Lord Yama takes away only our life, you take both our life as well as our money too"!

May we not become such inhospitable humans and may we do our best for all those who come into contact with us.

A judicious blend is required with a personalized and mindful approach to each individual, rather than the disease. Attempting to heal the individual with the disease, and not merely focusing on the disease; is a good motto to keep in mind at all times.

May we improve their life by the best of our efforts and may we always strive to have a balance between heart and head, between empathy and intelligence thus living Yoga as skill in action (karmasu koushalam) at all times.

May we all be true therapists, ones who care for our human brethren who are in the throes of suffering (duhkha).

May we enable them to attain as best as possible a state of health and wellbeing (sukha) through the living giving and life transforming art and science of Yoga.

Contents

CHAPTER 1

YOGA CHIKITSA: Attaining And Maintaining A Dynamic State Of Health

Yogacharya Dr. Ananda Balayogi Bhavanani
MBBS, PGDFH, PGDY, ADY, FIAY, C-IAYT, MD (AM), DSc (Yoga)
Director and Professor Yoga Therapy, Institute of
Salutogenesis and Complementary Medicine (ISCM)
Sri Balaji Vidyapeeth, Pondicherry, India.

Introduction

The art and science of Yoga is first and foremost a Moksha Shastra meant to facilitate the attainment of the final freedom, liberation or emancipation of Kaivalya. However one of the important by-products of the Yogic way of living is attainment of health and wellbeing. This is brought about by right-use-ness of the body, emotions and mind with awareness and consciousness. This must be understood to be as healthy a dynamic state that may be attained inspite of the individual's Sabija Karma that manifests as their genetic predispositions and the environment into which they are born. Yoga also helps us to maintain and sustain this dynamic state of health after it has been attained though disciplined self effort and conscious awareness of life itself.

Yogamaharishi Dr Swami Gitananda Giri Guru Maharaj, the visionary founder of Ananda Ashram at the International Centre for Yoga Education and Research (ICYER) in Pondicherry and one of the foremost authorities on Yoga in the past century, has explained the concept of Yoga Chikitsa (Yoga as a therapy) in the following lucid manner.

Yoga Chikitsa is virtually as old as Yoga itself, indeed, the 'return of mind that feels separated from the Universe in which it exists' represents the first Yoga therapy. Yoga Chikitsa could be termed as man's first attempt at unitive understanding of mind-emotions-physical distress and is the oldest holistic concept and therapy in the world.

To achieve this Yogic integration at all levels of our being, it is essential that we take into consideration the all encompassing multi dimensional aspects of Yoga that include the following: a healthy life nourishing diet, a healthy and natural environment, a wholistic lifestyle, adequate bodywork through Asanas, Mudras and Kriyas, invigorating breath work through the use of Pranayama and the production of a healthy thought process through the higher practices of Jnana Yoga and Raja Yoga.

Yogi Swatmarama in the Hathayoga Pradipika, one of the classical Yoga texts gives us the assurance:

"One who tirelessly practises Yoga attains success irrespective of whether they are young, old decrepit, diseased or weak". He gives us the guarantee that Yoga improves health of all alike and wards off disease, provided we properly abide by the rules and regulations (yuvaa vrddho ativriddho vaa vyaadhito durbalo pi vaa abhyaasaat siddhimaapnoti sarvayogeshvatandritah-Hathayoga Pradipika I:64).

YOGIC PERSPECTIVE ON HEALTH:

Yoga aims to enable the individual to attain and maintain a dynamic sukha sthanam that may be defined as a dynamic sense of physical, mental and spiritual well being. The Bhagavad Gita defines Yoga as samatvam meaning thereby that Yoga is equanimity at all levels (yogasthah kurukarmani sangam tyaktva dhananjaya siddiyasidhyoh samobutva samatvam yoga uchyate – Bhagavad Gita II: 48). This may be also understood as a perfect state of health wherein physical homeostasis and mental equanimity occur in a balanced and healthy harmony.

Yoga understands health and well being as a dynamic continuum of human nature and not a mere 'state' to be attained and maintained. The lowest point on the continuum with the lowest speed of vibration is that of death whereas the highest point with the highest vibration is that of immortality. In between these two extremes lie the states of normal health and disease. For many, their state of health is defined as that 'state' in which they are able to function without hindrance whereas in reality, health is part of our evolutionary process towards Divinity. The lowest point on the dynamic health continuum with lowest speed of vibration may be equated with lowest forms of life and mineral matter while the highest point with highest speed of vibration may be equated with Divinity.

Structural aspects of the human being: Yoga considers that we are not just the physical body but are of a multifold universal nature. Concepts of pancha kosha (fivefold aspects of our existence) and trisharira (threefold aspect of our bodily nature) help us understand our multi-dimensional real nature where health and result from a dynamic interaction at all levels of existence. At the level of the gross body, Yoga and Ayurveda consider that the human body is made up of seven substances. These sapta dhatus are rasa (chyle), rakta (blood), maamsa (flesh), medas (adipose), asthi (bone), majjaa (marrow) and sukra (semen). Both these ancient health sciences understand importance of tridosha (three humors) whose balance is vital for good health. Health is further also understood as harmony of prana vayus (major energies of physiological function), upa prana vayus (minor energies of physiological function) and stability of nadis (subtle energy channels) with proper function of all chakras (major energy centres that may be correlated to the psycho-neuro-immuno-endocrine axis).

Tridoshas and health: The tridosha theory of health and disease that developed during the late Vedic period (circa 1500-800 BC) is common to virtually all Indian systems of medicine. Tridosha concept has correlation with pancha mahabhutas (elements of the manifest universe) as well as triguna (inherent qualities of nature). Health is understood to be the balanced harmony of the three humours in accordance with individual predisposition while disease results from an imbalanced disharmony.

Qualities of physical health according to Yoga: The Yogic view of health is exemplified in Shvetaasvatara Upanishad where it is said that the first signs of entering Yoga are lightness of body, health, thirstlessness of mind, clearness of complexion, a beautiful voice, an agreeable odour and scantiness of excretions (laghutvam arogyam alolupatvam varnaprasadam svara sausthavam ca ganghas subho mootra pureesam Yoga pravrittim prathamam vadanti- Shvetaasvatara Upanishad: II-13).

The Hathayoga Pradipika echoes these qualities when Yogi Svatmarama says, "Slimness of body, lustre on face, clarity of voice, brightness of eyes, freedom from disease, control over seminal ejaculation, stimulation of gastric heat and purification of subtle energy channels are marks of success in Hathayoga" (vapuh krsatvam vadane prasannataa naadasputatvam nayane sunirmale arogataa bindujayogni diipanam naadiivishuddhir hatha siddhi lakshanam- Hathayoga Pradipika II-78).

In the Patanjala Yoga Darshan we find an excellent description of the attributes of bodily perfection (kaya sampat). It is said in Vibhuti Pada that perfection of body includes beauty, gracefulness, strength, and adamantine hardness (rupa lavanya bala vajra samhanana kaya sampat- Yoga Darshan III: 47). The effulgence that is characteristic of good health is also mentioned when it is said that deep concentration on samana (energy of digestion) leads to radiant effulgence (samana jayat jvalanam -Yoga Darshan III: 41).

Qualities of mental health according to Yoga: Yoga not only considers physical health but also more importantly mental health. Qualities of a mentally healthy person (stitha prajna) are enumerated in the Bhagavad Gita as follows:

- Beyond passion, fear and anger (veeta raga bhaya krodhah-BG II.56)
- Devoid of possessiveness and egoism (nirmamo nirahamkarah- BG -II.7)
- Firm in understanding and unbewildered (sthira buddhir asammudhah-BG - V.20)
- Engaged in doing good to all creatures (sarva bhutahiteratah- BG V.25)
- Friendly and compassionate to all (maitrah karuna eva ca- BG XII.13)
- Pure hearted and skilful without expectation (anapekshah sucir daksah- BG XII.16)

The central theme of Yoga is the golden mean, finding the middle path, a constant search for moderation and a harmonious homeostatic balance. Yoga is the "unitive impulse" of life, which always seeks to unite diverse streams into a single powerful force. Proper practice produces an inner balance of mind that remains stable and serene even in the midst of chaos. This ancient science shows its adherents a clear path to the "eye of the storm" and ensures a stability that endures within, even as the cyclone rages externally.

Qualities of spiritual health according to Yoga: The Bhagavad Gita delineates qualities of a spiritually healthy person in verses 1, 2 and 3 of chapter XVI. These include: fearlessness (abhayam), purity of inner being (sattva samshuddhih), steadfastness in the path of knowledge (jnanayoga vyavasthitih), charity (danam), self control (dama), spirit of sacrifice (yajna), self analysis (svadhyaya), disciplined life (tapa), uprightness (arjavam), non violence (ahimsa), truthfulness (satyam), freedom from anger (akrodhah), spirit of renunciation (tyagah), tranquillity (shanti), aversion to defamation (apaishunam), compassion to all living creatures (daya bhutesv), non covetedness (aloluptvam), gentleness (maardavam), modesty (hrir acaapalam), vigour (tejah), forgiveness (kshama), fortitude (dhritih), cleanliness of body and mind (saucam), freedom from malice (adroho), and absence of pride (naa timaanita).

Relationship between food and health: Yoga emphasizes the importance of not only eating the right type of food but also the right amount and with the right attitude. Importance of not eating alone, as well as preparation and serving of food with love are brought out in the Yogic scheme of right living. Guna (inherent nature) of food is taken into consideration to attain and maintain good health. Modern dietary science of diet can learn a lot from this ancient concept of classification of food according to inherent nature as it is a totally neglected aspect of modern diet. The great Tamil poet-saint Tiruvalluvar offers sane advice on right eating when he says, "He who eats after the previous meal has been digested, needs not any medicine." (marunthuena vaendaavaam yaakkaikku arundiyathu atrathu poatri unnin-Tirukkural 942). He also says that life in the body becomes a pleasure if we eat food to digestive measure (attraal alavuarinthu unga aghduudambu pettraan nedithu uikkum aaru-Tirukkural 943). He also invokes the Yogic concept of Mitahara by advising that "eating medium quantity of agreeable foods produces health and wellbeing" (maarupaaduillaatha undi marutthuunnin oorupaadu illai uyirkku -Tirukkural 943).

YOGIC METHODS TO ATTAIN AND MAINTAIN HEALTH:

The science of Yoga has numerous practical techniques as well as advice for proper life style in order to attain and maintain health and well being. Bahiranga practices such as yama, niyama, asana and pranayama help produce physical health while antaranga practices of dharana and dhyana work on producing mental health along with pratyahara. A detailed description of these techniques and their benefits on health is beyond the preview of this chapter but it will suffice to say here that Yoga works towards restoration of normalcy in all systems of the human body with special emphasis on the psycho-neuro-immuno-endocrine axis. In addition to its preventive and restorative capabilities, Yoga also aims at promoting positive health that will help us to tide over health challenges that occur during our lifetime. Just as we save money in a bank to tide over financial crises, so also we can build up our positive health balance to help us manage unforeseen health challenges with faster recovery and recuperation. This concept of positive health is one of Yoga's unique contributions to modern healthcare as Yoga has both a preventive as well as promotive role in the healthcare of our masses. It is also inexpensive and can be used in tandem with other systems of medicine in an integrated manner to benefit patients. In the Gheranda Samhita, a classical treatise on Hathayoga, the human body is likened to an unbaked clay pot that is incapable of holding the contents and dissolves when faced with the challenge of water. It is only through intense heat generated by practice of Yoga that the human body gets baked, making it fit to hold the Divine Spirit (aama kumbha ivaambhastho jeeryamanah sada gatah yoganalena samdahya ghata shuddhim samacaret- Gheranda Samhita I:8).

Tirumoolar has given numerous references to therapeutic benefits of Yoga for attaining and maintaining health in his monumental Tirumandiram. He emphasizes Swara Yoga concepts when he says, "If breath flow dominates in left nostril on Mondays, Wednesdays and Fridays no bodily harm can occur" (velliven thingal vilangum budanmoondrun thalli idatthe tayangume yaamaagil olliya kaayatthuk koona milaiyendru- Tirumandiram 791). He has further described the human body as the temple of the divine and stresses on the proper preservation of the body with reverence and care. (udambinai munnam izhukken drirunden udambinuk kulle yuruporul kanden udambule uttaman koilkon daan endru udambinai yaanirun thombugin drene –Tirumandiram 725). He has emphasized purification of internal organs to attain an imperishable body with perfect health (chuzhattrik kodukkave chuttik kazhiyunj chuzhattri malatthaik kamalatthaip poorithu uzhattrik kodukkum ubayam arivaarkku azhattrith thavirththudal anjana mame- Tirumandiram 726). According to Swami Kuvalayananda, founder of Kaivalyadhama, one of the oldest Yoga institutes in India, positive health does not mean mere freedom from disease but is a jubilant and energetic way of living and feeling that is the peak state of well being at all levels – physical, mental, emotional, social and spiritual. He says that one of the aims of Yoga is to encourage positive hygiene and health through development of inner natural powers of body and mind. In doing so, Yoga gives special attention to various eliminative processes and reconditions inherent powers of adaptation and adjustment of body and mind. Thus, the development of positive powers of adaptation and adjustment, inherent to the internal environment of man, helps him enjoy positive health and not just mere freedom from disease. He emphasizes that Yoga produces nadi shuddhi (purification of all channels of communication) and mala shuddhi (eradication of factors that disturb balanced working of body and mind).

According to Swami Kuvalayananda, Yoga helps cultivation of positive health through three integral steps:

1. Cultivation of correct psychological attitudes (maitri, karuna, mudita and upekshanam towards those who are suka, duhkha, punya and apunya),
2. Reconditioning of neuro-muscular and neuro-glandular system – in fact, the whole body – enabling it to withstand stress and strain better,
3. Laying great emphasis on appropriate diet conducive to such a peak state of health, and encouraging the natural processes of elimination through various processes of nadi shuddhi or mala shuddhi.

According to Yogacharini Meenakshi Devi Bhavanani, Director ICYER at Ananda Ashram in Pondicherry, Yoga has a step-by-step method for producing and maintaining perfect health at all levels of existence. She explains that social behaviour is first optimized through an understanding and control of the lower animal nature (pancha yama) and development and enhancement of the higher humane nature (pancha niyama). The body is then strengthened, disciplined, purified, sensitized, lightened, energized and made obedient to the higher will through asana. Universal pranic energy that flows through body-mind-emotions-spirit continuum is intensified and controlled through pranayama using breath control as a method to attain controlled expansion of the vital cosmic energy. The externally oriented senses are explored, refined, sharpened and made acute, until finally the individual can detach themselves from sensory impressions at will through pratyahara. The restless mind is then purified, cleansed, focused and strengthened through concentration (dharana). If these six steps are thoroughly understood and practiced then the seventh, dhyana or meditation (a state of union of the mind with the object of contemplation) is possible. Intense meditation produces samadhi, or the enstatic feeling of Union, Oneness with the Universe. This is the perfect state of integration or harmonious health.

YOGIC CONCEPTS OF DISEASE:

Vyadhi (disease) is considered one of the nine obstacles (antaraya) to integrative oneness of Yoga (samadhi) according to Maharishi Patanjali (Yoga Darshan I: 30). Patanjali also enumerates manifest symptoms such as duhkha (mental or physical pain), daurmanasya (sadness or dejection), angamejayatva (anxious tremor) and shvasa prashvasah (respiratory irregularities) as concomitant expressions of mental disturbances (Yoga Darshan I: 31). These antaraya are one of the major causes of disintegration (vyadhi) according to the late Dr ML Gharote, an eminent Yoga expert of Kaivalyadhama. He has described samadhi as the ideal state of health which is disturbed by the chitta vikshepa (disturbances in mind) due to the kleshas and antarayas. He has further also stated that mind is responsible for bondage and liberation as well as happiness and unhappiness. According to him the purpose of Yoga is to lessen the impact of these factors (klesha tanukaranam) and promote the state of integration (samadhi bhavanam). Maharishi Patanjali gives us a clue to control the mental agitation by advising us to concentrate on slow and deep flow of respiration to still the mind (prachchhardana vidharanabhyam va pranasya - Yoga Darshan I: 34). He also advises concentration on a painless inner state of luminosity to produce stability and tranquility (vishokava jyotishmati- Yoga Darshan I.36).

Patanjali has also explained the primary causation of stress based disorders through concept of pancha klesha (psychological afflictions). These are avidya (ignorance of the ultimate reality leading to bodily identification), asmita (a false sense of identification), raga-dwesha (addiction and aversion), abhinivesha (clinging on to life for fear of death), (avidya asmita raga dwesha abhinivesha kleshah -Yoga Darshan II: 3). Avidya as the root cause enables other kleshas to manifest in different forms from time to time. They may be dormant, attenuated, manifest or overpowering in their causation of pain and suffering. (avidya kshetram uttaresham prasupta tanu vicchinna udaranam- Yoga Darshan II: 4).

As a proponent of preventive medicine, he advises us to prevent that which can be prevented so as to avoid future pain and suffering (heyam duhkham anagatam -Yoga Darshan II: 16). This helps us to understand that disease is not something to be feared but is an indicator of where we have been erroneous in our lifestyle, thinking pattern or diet. When this is done with awareness and conscious self analysis is made, it can become an impetus for healthy change putting us back on the right track to a happier and healthier life. Suffering or duhkha can be a dynamic springboard in our evolution if we have the right attitude towards it and don't wallow in self pity.

Yoga helps train our whole process of thinking thus creating right attitudes for evolutionary growth, every moment of our life. The Yogic concept of health and disease enables us to understand that the cause of physical disorders stems from the seed in the mind and beyond. Adhi (the disturbed mind) is the cause and vyadhi (the physical disease) only the manifest effect in the Yogic scheme of things. By paying careful attention to personal history, one can nearly always trace origins of psychosomatic disease back to patterns of mental and emotional pressures. From the Yogic viewpoint of disease it can be seen that psychosomatic, stress related disorders appear to progress through four distinct phases. These can be understood as follows:

1. Psychic Phase: This phase is marked by mild but persistent psychological and behavioural symptoms of stress like irritability, disturbed sleep and other minor symptoms. This phase can be correlated with vijnanamaya and manomaya koshas. Yoga as a therapy is very effective in this phase.

2. Psychosomatic Phase: If the stress continues there is an increase in symptoms, along with the appearance of generalized physiological symptoms such as occasional hypertension and tremors. This phase can be correlated with manomaya and pranamaya koshas. Yoga as a therapy is very effective in this phase

3. Somatic Phase: This phase is marked by disturbed function of organs, particularly the target, or involved organ. At this stage one begins to identify the diseased state. This phase can be correlated with pranamaya and annamaya koshas. Yoga as a therapy is less effective in this phase and may need to be used in conjunction with other methods of treatment.

4. Organic Phase: This phase is marked by full manifestation of the diseased state, with pathological changes such as an ulcerated stomach or chronic hypertension, becoming manifest in their totality with their resultant complications. This phase can be correlated with the annamaya kosha as the disease has become fixed in the physical body. Yoga as a therapy has a palliative and quality of life improving effect in this phase. It does also produce positive emotional and psychological effects even in terminal and end of life situations.

Often, however, the early stages of the disease process are overlooked and the final stage is seen as an entity unto itself, having little relationship to one's living habits and patterns. This is because modern medicine only looks at the physical aspects and neglects effects of pancha kosha and trisharira on health and disease.

One of the major Indian concepts of disease causation is the imbalances of tridosha. This is found in numerous classical texts of Yoga and Ayurveda like Shiva Swarodaya, Sushruta Samhita, Charaka Samhita and Tirumandiram. According to the Dravidian poet-saint Tiruvalluvar, disease results from tridosha imbalance (miginum kuraiyinum noiseyyum noolor valimudhalaa enniya moondru -Tirukkural 941). Vata is the energy of the body that moves like the wind and causes flow in the body. It may be related to the nervous system as well as joints that enable us to move. Pitta is related to bilious secretion and is the cause of heat in the body. It is the energy of catabolism that is essential for digestion. Kapha is the glue that holds everything together and is the energy of anabolism helping generative and regenerative processes.

According to Mark Halpern, Founder-Director, California College of Ayurveda, USA the tridosha fluctuate constantly. As they move out of balance, they affect particular areas of our bodies in characteristic ways. When vata is out of balance—typically in excess—we are prone to diseases of the large intestines, like constipation and gas, along with diseases of nervous system, immune system, and joints. When pitta is in excess, we are prone to diseases of the small intestines, like diarrhoea, along with diseases of the liver, spleen, thyroid, blood, skin, and eyes. When kapha is in excess, we are prone to diseases of the stomach and lungs, most notably mucous conditions, along with diseases of water metabolism, such as swelling.

Yoga Vashista, a classical Yoga text describes causation and manifestation of disease in an admirable manner. It describes both psychosomatic as well as non-psychosomatic ailments. It attributes all psychic disturbances and physical ailments to the fivefold elements namely the pancha mahabhuta in a manner similar to other systems of Indian medicine. Samanya adhija vyadhi are described as those arising from day-to-day causes while sara adhija vyadhi is the essential disease of being caught in the birth –rebirth cycle that can be understood in modern terms as congenital diseases. The former can be corrected by day-to-day remedial measures such as medicines and surgery whereas the sara adhija vyadhi doesn't cease until knowledge of the self (atma jnana) is attained. The Guru Stotra from the

Vishvasaaraatantra also takes a similar line in saying that the ultimate 'wisdom of the self' gained through the Guru destroys karmic bondages from many births (anekajanma samprapta karma bandha vidhahine atmajnana pradanena tasmai srigurave namah-Guru Stotra, verse 9). It is interesting to note that traditional Indian thought views the very occurrence of birth on this planet as a disease and a source of suffering! Tiruvalluvar reiterates this when he says, "It is knowledge of the ultimate truth that removes the folly of birth" (pirappu ennum pedaimai neenga chirappu ennum chem porul kaanbadhu arivu- Tirukkural 358)

Yoga understands that physical ailments that are not of a psychosomatic nature can be easily managed with surgery, medication, prayers, douches and lifestyle modifications as required. Various Yoga techniques may also be used to help correct the physical ailments and restore health with regeneration, recuperation and rehabilitation as necessary. Accident prevention is an important benefit of a Yoga life, for better alertness, reflexes and physical condition enables one to prevent accidents as well as avoid getting traumatized both physically and mentally by such occurrences.

Yoga Vashista gives an elaborate description of the mechanism by which psychosomatic disorders occur. Mental confusion leads to agitation of prana (life force) and haphazard flow along nadis resulting in depletion of energy and / or clogging up of these channels of vital energy. This leads to disturbance in the physical body with disturbances of metabolism, excessive appetite and improper functioning of the entire digestive system. Natural movement of food through the digestive tract is arrested giving rise to numerous physical ailments. We need to remember that this text is many thousands of years old whereas the concept of psychosomatic disorders in modern medicine has only been realized and accepted in recent times. Our ancients had great inner vision and it is up to us to realize their dreams and understand the great message they have left for humanity.

According to Shivaswarodaya, a classical text on Swara Yoga, disease develops when swara (smooth and regular air flow) in the nostrils do not adhere to their fixed timings and days. Normally swara flows in the nostrils in a certain pattern according to phases of the lunar cycle. It is also said that in case a disease develops due to erroneous functioning of swara, then a correction of that malfunctioning can cure that disease. The use of different techniques is also advocated for changing swara to relive various disorders.

Yogamaharishi Dr Swami Gitananda Giri, founder of Ananda Ashram at Pondicherry has written extensively about the relationship between health and disease. He says, "Yoga views the vast proliferation of psychosomatic diseases as a natural outcome of stress and strain created by desire fostered by modern propaganda and abuse of the body condoned on all sides even by religion, science and philosophy. Add to this the synthetic "junk food" diet of modern society and you have the possibility of endless disorders developing…even the extinction of man by his own ignorance and misdeeds".

He explains the root cause of disease as follows. "Yoga, a wholistic, unified concept of oneness, is adwaitam or non-dual in nature. It suggests happiness, harmony and ease. Dis-ease is created when duality or dwaitam arises in the human mind. This false concept of duality has produced all conflicts of human mind and the vast list of human disorders. Duality (dis-ease) is the primary cause of man's downfall. Yoga helps return man to his pristine, whole nature. All diseases, maladies, tensions, are manifestations of divisions of what should be man's complete nature, the atman or 'Self'. This 'Self' is "ease". A loss of "ease" creates "dis-ease". Duality is the first insanity, the first disease, the unreasonable thought that "I am different from the whole…. I am unique. I am me." The ego is a manifestation of disease. Only a distorted ego could feel alone, suffer from "the lonely disease", in a Universe, a Cosmos totally filled with the 'Self'. It is interesting that one of the oldest words for man is "insan". Man is "insane". A return to sanity, "going sane," is the subject of real Yoga sadhana and Yoga abhyasa. Yoga chikitsa is one of the methods to help insane man back onto the path of sanity. A healthy man or woman may be known by the term-Yogi". A very strongly worded yet very true statement indeed from the Lion of Pondicherry!

APPLICATION OF YOGA AS A THERAPY:

The Tridosha theory of health and disease that developed during the late Vedic period is common to virtually all traditional Indian systems of medicine. Health is understood to be the balanced harmony of the three humours in accordance with individual predisposition while disease results from an imbalanced disharmony. Tirumandiram of Tirumoolar, the 3000 versed Tamil treatise by the Dravidian saint has prescribed the practice of Yoga at different times of day to relieve disorders arising from Tridosha imbalances. According to him, practice of Yoga at dusk relieves Kapha, practice at noon relieves Vata and practice in morning relieves Pitta disorders (anjanam pondruda laiyaru mandiyile vanjaga vatha marumaddi yaanatthir senjiru kaalaiyir seithidir pittarum nanjara sonnom naraithirai naasame –Tirumandiram 727).

To live a healthy life it is important to do healthy things and follow a healthy lifestyle. The modern world is facing a pandemic of lifestyle disorders that require changes to be made consciously by individuals themselves. Yoga places great importance on a proper and healthy lifestyle whose main components are:

1. Achar – Yoga stresses the importance of healthy activities such as exercise and recommends Asana, Pranayama and Kriyas on a regular basis. Cardio-respiratory health is one of the main by-products of such healthy activities.
2. Vichar – Right thoughts and right attitude towards life is vital for well being. A balanced state of mind is obtained by following the moral restraints and ethical observances (Yama-Niyama). As Mahatma Gandhi said, "there is enough in this world for everyone's need but not enough for any one person's greed".
3. Ahar – Yoga emphasises need for a healthy, nourishing diet that has an adequate intake of fresh water along with a well balanced intake of fresh food, green salads, sprouts, unrefined cereals and fresh fruits. It is important to be aware of the need for a Satwic diet, prepared and served with love and affection.
4. Vihar – Proper recreational activities to relax body and mind are

essential for good health. This includes proper relaxation, maintaining quietude of action-speech-thoughts and group activities wherein one loses the sense of individuality. Karma Yoga is an excellent method for losing the sense of individuality and gaining a sense of universality.

5. Vyavahar – Healthy relationships that enable health and wellness to manifest through positive peer support groups and satsangha.

The application of Yoga as a therapy can be correlated with the Pancha Koshas (the five aspects of our existence) and various Yoga practices may be used as therapeutic interventions at different levels in this respect.

• At the Annamaya Kosha (anatomical level of existence) Jattis (simple units of movements), Mudras (gestures for energy generation and conservation), Kriyas (structured movements), Asanas (steady and comfortable postures) along with the dietary modifications are useful.

• At the Pranamaya Kosha (physiological level of existence) Shat Karmas (cleansing actions), various Pranayamas, development of breath awareness and working on breath-movement coordination with emphasis on balancing Pranic energy is to be done. Work on reenergizing and integrating the energies of the Pancha Prana and Upa Prana Vayus needs to be done at this level.

• At the Manomaya Kosha (psychological level of existence) there are numerous practices such as Trataka (concentrated gaze), Dharana (concentration), Dhyana (meditation), Japa and Japa-Ajapa practices that are useful. Various aspects of concentration such as the Mandala Dharana and other Yoga Drishti techniques are also available in the Gitananda tradition for this purpose. An awareness of all aspects of the Antah Karanas needs to be developed at this level.

• When trying to deal with the Vijnanamaya Kosha (intellectual level of existence) Swadhyaya (self analysis), Satsangha (lectures and spiritually uplifting exchange) along with the wonderful Jnana Yoga and Raja Yoga relaxation and concentration practices of Yoga are useful. We must remember that according to Swamiji, we thankfully cannot disturb the Vijnanamaya and Anandamaya Koshas! However what can happen is that we get the other three bodies out of sync with the higher two and so suffer consequences of such ignorant actions.

- To understand and work with the Anandamaya Kosha (our universal level of existence) it is important to loose sense of the limited individuality. Learning to implement principles of Karma Yoga (Yoga as skilled action performed without expectation) and following the principle of action in relaxation help us to achieve a sense of joy in all activities. A realization that we live in a blissful universe and that all life is joy is to be brought about in this intervention through use of Bhakti Yoga, Karma Yoga and other aspects like Bhajana, Yogic counselling and Satsangha

Yoga is basically a preventive life-science and hence Yogic counselling is a vital component of Yoga Chikitsa when dealing with all lifestyle disorders. The counselling process is not a 'one off' matter but is a continuous process that starts from the very first visit and continues with every session at different levels. Helping the patients understand their condition, finding the root cause of the problem and creating a healthy opportunity for them to change themselves, is the Dharma of the therapist. My beloved Ammaji (Yogacharini Meenakshi Devi Bhavanani) has defined Dharma as doing the right thing for the right person at the right place and at the right time in the right manner. It may take many months before we start to witness benefits of these Yogic lifestyle changes and Yoga Chikitsa practices. We must continue to motivate the patient (and ourselves too!) to keep up their (our) efforts without allowing any slackening to occur.

PRINCIPLES OF YOGA CHIKITSA:

When we set out to practice Yoga Chikitsa it is vital that we are conversant with important principles of this unique system of healthy living. One of the outcomes of Yoga practice is attainment of health. This implies as healthy a state that may be attained in spite of our Sabija Karma that manifests in this lifetime as our genetic predispositions and the environment we are born into. Yoga also helps maintain and sustain this dynamic state of health after it has been attained though self effort. We must not however forget that it is often actually more challenging to maintain this state than to attain it in the first place. Ask any World No.1 Sports Champion and they will testify to this inherent truth that applies to sports as well as to life itself.

1. BECOME AWARE OF YOUR BODY, EMOTIONS AND MIND: Without awareness there cannot be health or healing. Awareness of body implies conscious body work that needs to be synchronized with breath to qualify as a psychosomatic technique of health and healing. Psychosomatic disorders that are the bane of the modern world cannot be tackled without awareness.

2. IMPROVE YOUR DIETARY HABITS: Most disorders are directly or indirectly linked to improper dietary patterns that need to be addressed in order to find a permanent solution to the health challenge. One of the most important lifestyle changes that needs be implemented in management of any lifestyle disorder is diet.

3. RELAX YOUR WHOLE BODY: Relaxation is most often all that most patients need in order to improve their physical condition. Stress is the major culprit and may be the causative, aggravating, or precipitating factor in so many psychosomatic disorders. Doctors are often found telling their patients to relax, but never tell them how to do it! The relaxation part of every Yoga session is most important for it is during it that benefits of practices done in the session seep into each and every cell producing rest, rejuvenation, reinvigoration and reintegration.

4. SLOW DOWN YOUR BREATH MAKING IT QUIET AND DEEP: Rapid, uncontrolled, irregular breathing is a sign of ill health whereas slow, deep and regular controlled breathing is a sign of health. Breath is the link between body and mind and is the agent of physical, physiological and mental unification. When the breath is slowed down the metabolic processes also are slowed and anabolic activities begin the process of healing and rebuilding. If breath is calm, mind is calm and life is long!

5. CALM DOWN YOUR MIND AND FOCUS IT INWARDLY: The mind is as disturbed as a drunken monkey bitten by a scorpion say our scriptures. To bring that wayward agitated mind under control, and take it on a journey into our inner being is fundamental in finding a way out of the 'disease maze' in which we are entangled like a fly in the spider's web. Breath work is the base on which this mind training can occur and hence much importance needs to be given to Pranayama and Pratyahara in Yoga Chikitsa. It is only after this that concentration practices leading to meditation can have any use. Just sitting and thinking about something is not meditation!

6. IMPROVE THE FLOW OF HEALING 'PRANIC LIFE ENERGY': Improve the flow of Healing 'Pranic Life Energy' to all parts of your body, especially to those diseased parts, thus relaxing, regenerating and reinvigorating yourself. Prana is life and without it there cannot be healing. The various Prana Vayus that are energies driving different physiological functions of the body need to be understood and applied as per needs of the patient. In patients of digestive disorders, focus must be on the Samana Vayu whereas in pelvic conditions it needs to be on Apana Vayu.

7. FORTIFY YOURSELF AGAINST OMNIPRESENT STRESSORS: Decrease your stress level by fortifying yourself against the various omnipresent stressors in your life: when face to face with the innumerable thorns in a forest, you may either choose to spend all your time picking them up one by one while others continue falling or choose to wear a pair of shoes and walk through the forest. The difference is in attitude. Choosing the right attitude can change everything and bring about a resolution of the problem by healing the core. Stress is more about how you react to the stressor than about the stressor itself!

8. INCREASE YOUR SELF RELIANCE AND SELF CONFIDENCE: Life is full of challenges that are there only to make us stronger and better. The challenges should be understood as opportunities for change and faced with confidence. We must understand we have the inner power to overcome each and every challenge that is thrown at us by life.

The Divine is not a sadist to give us challenges that are beyond our capacity!

9. FACILITATE NATURAL EMANATION OF WASTES: Facilitate the natural emanation of waste from your body by the practice of Yoga Shuddhi Kriyas such as Dhauti, Basti and Neti. Accumulation and stagnation of waste materials either in inner or outer environment always causes problems. Yogic cleaning practices held to wash out the impurities (Mala Shodhana) helping the process of regeneration and facilitating healing.

10. TAKE RESPONSIBILITY FOR YOUR OWN HEALTH: Remember that ultimately it is "YOU" who are responsible for your own health and well being and must take the initiative to develop positive health to tide you over challenging times of ill health. Yoga fixes responsibility for our health squarely upon our own shoulders. If we do healthy things we are healthy and if we do unhealthy things we become sick. No use complaining that we are not well when we have been the cause of our problem. As Swamiji Gitananda Giri would say, "You don't have problems-you are the problem!"

11. HEALTH AND HAPPINESS ARE YOUR BIRTHRIGHT: Health and happiness are your birthright, claim them and develop them to your maximum potential. This message of Swamiji is a firm reminder that the goal of human existence is not health and happiness but is Moksha (liberation). Most people today are so busy trying to find health and happiness that they forget why they are here in the first place. Yoga helps us regain our birthrights and attain the goal of human life.

SCIENTIFIC BASIS OF USING YOGA AS A THERAPY:

Numerous studies have been done in the past few decades on psycho-physiological and biochemical changes occurring following practice of Yoga. A few clinical trials have also been done that have shown promise despite Yoga not being ideally suited for the scientific gold standard of 'double-blind' clinical trials.

It is virtually impossible for subjects to be taught Yoga without their knowing it is Yoga! The difficulty of finding right methods and apparatus to study higher aspects of Yoga is still to be overcome as there doesn't seem to be much money in it and as we know, money makes the world go round!

Some of the researched benefits that are quite well proven are given below to facilitate an understanding of how Yoga works at least at the physical level though we are yet to research and understand subtler effects of Yoga.

- PHYSIOLOGICAL BENEFITS OF YOGA: It has been found that Yoga produces stable autonomic nervous system equilibrium, with a tendency toward parasympathetic nervous system dominance rather than the usual stress-induced sympathetic nervous system dominance. This is of great potential in psychosomatic stress related illness abounding in populations worldwide. Cardiovascular and cardio-respiratory efficiency increases. Heart rate and blood pressure decrease implying a better state of relaxation leading to reduced load on the heart. Respiratory rate decreases with improved respiratory efficiency. The amplitude and smoothness of respiration increases, along with all parameters of pulmonary function such as tidal volume, vital capacity and breath-holding time. EEG - alpha waves increase. Theta, delta, and beta waves also increase during various stages of meditation. Gastrointestinal function and endocrine function normalizes with improvement in excretory functions. Musculoskeletal flexibility and joint range of motion increase. Posture improves with improvement in strength, resiliency and endurance. Body weight normalizes and sleep improves with increased energy levels and the immunity increases with improved ability of pain tolerance.

- PSYCHOLOGICAL BENEFITS OF YOGA: It has been found that somatic and kinesthetic awareness increase with better self-acceptance and self-actualization. There is better social adjustment with decrease in anxiety, depression and hostility. Psychomotor functions such as grip strength, balance, dexterity and fine motor skills, eye hand coordination and reaction time, steadiness and depth perception, and the integrated functioning of body parts improve. Mood improves and subjective well-being increases while cognitive functions such as attention, concentration, memory, and learning efficiency improve.

- BIOCHEMICAL EFFECTS OF YOGA: The biochemical profile improves, indicating an anti-stress and antioxidant effect which is important in the prevention of degenerative diseases. There are decreased levels of blood glucose, total white blood cell count, total cholesterol, Triglycerides, LDL and VLDL. At the same time it has been reported that there are increased levels of: HDL cholesterol, ATPase, hematocrit, hemoglobin, thyroxin, lymphocytes, vitamin C and total serum protein following Yoga.

THERAPEUTIC MODALITIES OF YOGA CHIKITSA:

There are numerous therapeutic modalities used in the application of Yoga as a therapy. Pujya Swamiji Gitananda Giri has enumerated 52 aspects of Yoga Chikitsa in an encyclopedic manner. His exposition of Yoga Chikitsa is unparalleled yet this is a small attempt of mine to put some of these ancient ideas into a modern context for us all to work together towards a harmonious and healthy world. Some of the commonly used modalities are as following:

- PHYSICAL THERAPIES: Asanas (static postures), Kriyas (systematic and rationale movements), Mudras (seals of neuromuscular energy) and Bandhas (locks for neuromuscular energy) gently stretch and strengthen the musculoskeletal system in a healthy manner. They improve mobility and flexibility of the different joints and groups of muscles. There is also concomitant improvement in the systemic function such as respiration, circulation, digestion and elimination. A general sense of health and well being is also promoted by these aspects of Yoga that help release feel good hormones like endorphins and encephalin.

- EMOTIONAL THERAPIES: Swadhyaya (introspectional self analysis), Pranayama (techniques of vital energy control), Pratyahara (sensory withdrawal), Dharana (intense concentration), Dhyana (meditational oneness) and Bhajana (devotional music) stabilize emotional turmoil and relieve stress and mental fatigue. They bring about an excellent sense of emotional balance that is vital for good health. Group work such as this is important to achieve proper emotional balance that is essential to good health.

- DEVELOPMENT OF PROPER PSYCHOLOGICAL ATTITUDES: Yoga encourages us to step back and take an objective view of our habitual patterns of behaviour and thoughts. This enables us to cope better with situations that normally put our bodies and minds under strain. Patanjali emphasized the need to develop the following qualities in order to become mentally balanced humane beings: Vairagya (detached, dispassionate attitude), Chitta Prasadanam (acceptance of the Divine Will), Maitri (friendliness towards those who are at peace with themselves), Karuna (compassion for the suffering), Mudita (cheerfulness towards the virtuous) and Upekshanam (indifference and avoidance of the evil) etc. Adoption of the right attitude is one of the most important aspects of Yoga as a therapy and if this is not done it is again more or less Yogopathy and not Yoga Chikitsa.

- MENTAL THERAPIES: There are a great many Jnana and Raja Yoga techniques of relaxation and visualization that are useful. Other practices such as Trataka (concentrated gaze), Pranayama, Pratyahara, Dharana as well as Dhyana may also be utilized. Relaxation is a central element in Yoga as it is the body's own way of recharging its cells and helps to ease physical, emotional and mental tensions.

- SPIRITUAL THERAPIES: Swadhyaya, Satsangha (spiritual gathering seeking knowledge of the reality), Bhajana sessions and Yogic counseling are important aspects of Yogic therapy that are often neglected in favor of physical therapies alone. It is important to help patients understand their inner spiritual nature and realize that "Oneness" is health whereas "Duality" is disease. We cannot remain lonely, depressed and diseased if we realize that we are part of this bountiful and wholesome, wonderful, happy and healthy Universe.

- PREVENTIVE AND REHABILITATIVE THERAPIES: Yoga has numerous preventive benefits especially when it is started early in childhood.

It helps in prevention of accidents by increasing awareness as well as agility. Improved immunity helps in preventing infectious and contagious diseases. The added benefit of starting early is that the person knows the technique so that they can do it if needed at a later stage in life. Psychosomatic, stress related and lifestyle disorders may be effectively prevented by adoption of a Yogic way of life. Yoga also offers rehabilitative therapies for most musculoskeletal conditions as well as in recovery for debilitating illnesses. The practice of Yoga also goes a long way towards prevention of disability and improving quality of life in numerous chronic conditions.

- PAIN RELIEF THERAPIES: Yoga is a useful addition to the pain relief therapies as it improves pain tolerance and provides an improved quality of life. It can be safely said that Yoga helps us endure conditions that it may not be able to cure. This is vital in end of life situations where it is important that the patient has a sense of improved quality of life during their end days. Yoga can also benefit caretakers of such terminal patients who are under great stress themselves.

The right-use-ness of these modalities according to condition and needs of patients will enable us to strike at the root cause of the disease and by correcting its origin. If this is done properly, the manifestation of the disease corrects itself and health and harmony can manifest once again.

YOGIC METHODS OF DIAGNOSIS:

When we start to use the art and science of Yoga as a therapy (Yoga Chikitsa) it is important that we realise the basic fact that Yoga has its own system of diagnosis and health evaluation. Please don't forget that the mere use of Yoga techniques to suppress symptoms is Yogopathy!

The twelve diagnostic methods (dwadasha rogalakshna anukrama) have been very well described by Yogamaharishi Dr Swami Gitananda Giri, founder of Ananda Ashram at Pondicherry, India and one of the foremost authorities on Yoga in the 20th century as a method of self-analysis (swadhyaya) that enables not only the therapist to understand the patient better but also enables at the same time the patient to understand themselves better too. This may then stimulate the patients themselves to make a sincere and dedicated attempt to regain their lost health, happiness and wholeness through unitive methods. This is a "win-win" situation and benefits all!

The twelve major methods of diagnosis used in yoga that have been described by Pujya Swamiji include:

1. Triguna: This is most important as a person of a tamasic (dull and lazy) nature needs to be treated differently than rajasic (overactive) and sattwic (calm and composed) types. Western medicine treats everyone "democratically the same" and turns simple toxicity into permanent sickness. The trigunic nature must first be evaluated to bring about self-healing in a patient. The more sensitive and evolved the person, the more sensitive must be the treatment.

2. Tridosha: Without evaluating patients according to their dosha, modern medicine dries up the kapha, increases chemical poisoning and produces pressure conditions that are all chronic disorders, while the original dosha imbalances may be easily rectified and balanced.

3. Trivasana: The psychological background to one's personal nature represents personal propensities that bind us to the wheel of birth and rebirth. Lokha vasana (attachment to one's position in life), jnana vasana (attachment to one's level of education and knowledge) and deha vasana (hang-ups and attachments to the body). These may be considered to be the most ingrained of all human conditions.

4. Prana: One must determine which of the prana vayu is active or recessive, and which upa prana vayu is shut down, inactive, or recessive. Improper functioning of the various prana vayu leads to various conditions depending on the vayu involved. For example, if it is the samana vayu, then digestion is affected whereas the excretory function is affected in apana vayu malfunction. Loss of prana is death whereas disease is the manifestation of pranic malfunction.

5. Abhyasa: A disciplined patient can be trusted to carry out directions,

while those who are undisciplined will be difficult patients, disobeying injunctions about life, transgressing body laws, and therefore, will remain disturbed, negative and ill. A disciplined person is seldom ill and is usually suffering only from ignorance or avidya. When truth is revealed they will immediately follow the truth. Most real Gurus will refuse to accept students unless they are disciplined but Yoga therapists don't always really have that choice!

6. Jiva Karma: A healthy lifestyle is one where there is proper adherence to yama-niyama, the system of morality and ethics, as expounded by Maharishi Patanjali. Disobedience or lack of discretion in following these moral and ethical precepts are the cause of much sickness, pain, suffering and violence. A moral and ethical life is necessary for attaining and maintaining good health.

7. Chetana: The quality of thought of the individual matters! Are the patient's thoughts idealistic, positive, and outgoing? Or are they lacking in ideals, reserved and negative? Thought is the cause of all body action and this is the rationale behind adhi-vyadhi, the Yogic concept of psycho-somatics. The Christ Yogi said, "As above, so below"- As we think so also we become. Nowdays we are faced with dangerous vyadhi-adhi, somato – psychic conditions where diseased condition of the body in turn produces mental disturbances. Talk of the tail wagging the dog!

8. Vacha: Much can be diagnosed from the way a person speaks, how they pronounce and enunciate language and how they deliver the "power of sound in speech". Refined speech should be met with refined results. Crude and rough speech elicits crude and rough response. An understanding of the different regions related to production of sound such as the nabhi (navel), hridaya (heart), kanta (throat), rasana (tongue), nasa (nose) etc are essential to be able to utilise this method properly. Saint Thiyagaraja, the great south Indian music composer has delineated these regions and their importance in producing the seven sacred notes of Indian music in his krithi (song) shobillu saptaswara (the seven beautiful heavenly notes of music).

9. Ahara: As food plays an important part in health or sickness, dietary habits must be examined in great detail. It is universally understood that a meat-eating diet is destructive, while a vegetarian diet is more conducive to good health, emotional equilibrium and unitive evolution. Junk foods especially must be curtailed. Tiruvalluvar, the great Dravidian poet-saint has emphasized the link between overeating and disease by saying, "the one who eats on an empty stomach gets health while with the greedy glutton abides ill-health" (izhivu arindhu unbaankan inbampol nirkum kazhiper iraiyaankan noi- Tirukkural 946). He offers sane advice on right eating when he says, "He who eats after the previous meal has been digested, needs not any medicine." (marunthuena vaendaavaam yaakkaikku arundiyathu atrathu poatri unnin-Tirukkural 942). He also invokes the Yogic concept of Mitahara by advising that "eating medium quantity of agreeable foods produces health and wellbeing" (maarupaaduillaatha undi marutthuunnin oorupaadu illai uyirkku -Tirukkural 943).

10. Viparita Buddhi. There is no possibility of good health for a person who deliberately misuses tobacco, alcohol and illicit drugs. Other habits like over eating or under eating, over exercise and under exercise as well as sexual abuses must also be considered. Viparita Buddhi is considered one of the final steps on the road to self induced disaster as made clear by the common statement "vinashkale viparita buddhi" (when the end is near the intelligence is lost).

11. Jiva Vritti: Considerations such as periodicity of the nasal cycle, number of breaths per minute (whether deep or shallow, whether sectional or complete), periodicity and rate of the heart, blood pressure, regularity of passing urine and emptying of bowels etc are classified in this category.

12. Sankalpa: Aspirations of the individual which may only involve a desire to be well must also be examined. What are the beliefs of the patient? Are they negative or positive? High or low? Are they idealistic enough to accept help, suggestions, and spiritual advice, or are they the type who rejects positive help. It is most often the case that the one who

accepts is a ready listener, and usually follows up with direct actions leading to betterment of health and attainment of well being.

CURRENT SITUATION OF YOGA THERAPY:

Modern Yoga therapy seems to have lost touch with the real essence of Yoga. The art and science of Yoga aims to help us regain our psycho-physiological balance, by removing the root cause of the disharmony (dukkasamyogaviyogam yogasamjnitham – Bhagavad Gita VI: 23). Yet, as Yoga therapists, unless we aim to correct the manifest psycho-somatic disassociation as well as the underlying ignorant, jaundiced perception of reality in the individual, we are really not practicing Yoga Chikitsa.

Managing and suppressing the manifest symptoms with Yoga techniques is just as good or bad as modern Allopathic medicine that focuses primarily on symptomatic management without ever getting close to the "real" cause of most disorders. How many doctors look at the emotional and psychological issues that are the primary cause of the problem in so many of their patients? Remember, the concept of psychosomatics is not older than a hundred years in modern medicine and any doctor talking about 'mind affecting body' disease a couple of hundred years ago risked getting labelled a quack and may have even been crucified at the altar of science! When today we find our Yoga therapists making the same mistake in merely treating manifesting symptoms without remedying the 'real' cause, I prefer to call it Yogopathy! It may be useful for many but please do understand that it loses the special wholesome nature of Yoga and is no longer Yoga Chikitsa anymore.

An example of this Yogopathy trend is when we use Shavasana to manage patients of hypertension quoting research that has shown that Shavasana reduces blood pressure. We seem happy just to bring the blood pressure down for the time being! Real Yoga Chikitsa would try to look for the primary cause of the patient's hypertension and try to tackle that along with Shavasana for symptomatic management. Without an attempt to remedy the root cause, it remains merely Yogopathy.

Another common example is of using the left nostril Chandra Nadi Pranayama to lower the blood sugar or using the right nostril Surya Nadi Pranayama to relieve brochospasm without looking for the real cause of the patient's diabetes or asthma. When we do this, how are we any different than the modern doctors who prescribe anti-diabetic and sympatho-mimetic agents for these patients? Where is the real Yoga in this type of therapy? Where is the effort to find and deal with the primary cause? Without a positive change in attitude or lifestyle, can it be Yoga Chikitsa?

In the application of Yoga Chikitsa it is vital that we take into consideration all the following aspects that are part of an integrated approach to the problem. These include a healthy life nourishing diet, a healthy and natural environment, a wholistic lifestyle, adequate bodywork through Asanas, Mudras and Kriyas, invigorating breath work through the use of Pranayama and the production of a healthy thought process through the higher practices of Jnana and Raja Yoga.

Extensive research on Yoga being done all over the world has shown promise with regard to various disorders and diseases indicating scientifically the feasibility of them being amiable to the application of Yoga as a therapy. However we must remember to try and deal with the root cause for if not, we are going to only be practicing YOGOPATHY and not Yoga Chikitsa! As Yoga Chikitsa starts to be introduced into mainstream health care, we must not fall into the dangerous trap of claiming that Yoga is a miracle that can cure everything under the sun for that "puts off" the modern medical community more than anything. They then develop a stiff resistance to Yoga instead of becoming more open to this life giving and health restoring science. As the use of Yoga Chikitsa in medical centers is still in its infancy we must be cautious about the after-effects we may produce by our conscious and unconscious thoughts, words and actions. Better to err on the side of caution than be true to the adage, "fools rush in where angels fear to tread".

I am not downplaying the potentiality of Yoga for it DOES have a role in virtually each and every condition. We must however realize that though Yoga can improve the condition of nearly every patient, it doesn't necessarily translate into words such as cure. Modern medicine doesn't have a cure for most conditions and so when Yoga therapists use such words, it creates a negative image that does more harm than good.

I would like to reiterate at this point the need of the modern age which is to have an integrated approach towards all forms of therapy. We must try to integrate concepts of Yoga in coordination and collaboration with other systems of medicine such as Allopathy, Ayurveda, Siddha and Naturopathy. Physiotherapy, osteopathy and chiropractic practices may be also used with the Yoga Chikitsa as required. Don't forget that advice on diet and adoption of a healthy lifestyle is very important irrespective of the mode of therapy employed for the patient.

Yoga can for sure, help regain the ease we had lost earlier through dis-ease (as implied by sthira sukham asanam- Yoga Darshan II: 46). It can also enable us to attain a dynamic state of mental equanimity (samatvam yoga uchyate- Bhagavad Gita II: 48) where the opposites cease to affect us any

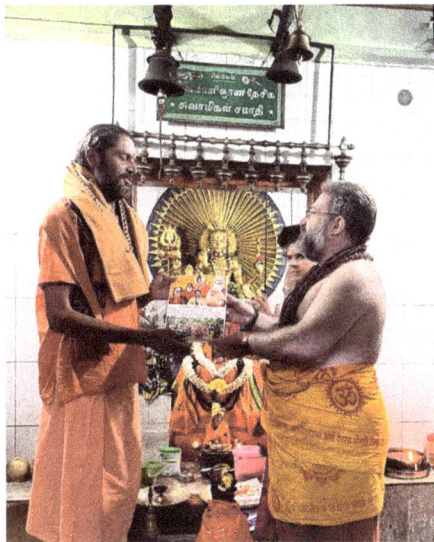

more (tato dwandwa anabhigatha- Yoga Darshan II: 48). This enables us to move from a state of illness and disease to one of health and wellbeing that ultimately allows us to move from a lower animal nature to a higher human nature and finally reach the highest Divine Nature that is our birthright.

RECOMMENDED READING:

1. A Primer of Yoga Theory. Dr Ananda Balayogi Bhavanani. Dhivyananda Creations, Iyyanar Nagar, Pondicherry. 2008. www.rishiculture.org

2. Back issues of International Journal of Yoga Therapy. Journal of the International Association of Yoga Therapists, USA. www.iayt.org

3. Back issues of Yoga Life, Monthly Journal of ICYER at Ananda Ashram, Pondicherry. www.icyer.com

4. Back issues of Yoga Mimamsa. Journal of Kaivalyadhama, Lonavla, Maharashtra.

5. Four Chapters on Freedom. Commentary on Yoga Sutras of Patanjali by Swami Satyananda Saraswathi, Bihar School of Yoga, Munger, India. 1999

6. Srimad Bhagavad Gita by Swami Swarupananda. Advaita Ashrama, Kolkata. 2007

7. The Supreme Yoga: Yoga Vashista. Swami Venkatesananda. Motilal Banarsidass Publishers Pvt Ltd. Delhi.2007

8. Tiruvalluvar on Yogic Concepts. Meena Ramanathan, Aarogya Yogalayam, Venkateswara Nagar, Saram, Pondicherry-13.2007

9. Yoga for health and healing. Dr Ananda Balayogi Bhavanani. Dhivyananda Creations, Iyyanar Nagar, Pondicherry. 2008. www.rishiculture.org

10. Yoga: Step-by-Step. A 52 lesson correspondence course by Dr Swami Gitananda Giri. Ananda Ashram at ICYER, Pondicherry. www.ciyer.com

11. Yoga Therapy Notes. Dr Ananda Balayogi Bhavanani. Dhivyananda Creations, Iyyanar Nagar, Pondicherry. 200w

CHAPTER 2
by Yogachariya Jnandev Giri
The three bodies and five sheaths (Pancha - Kosha) concept of Yoga

Yoga Darshan explains that our living existential body is made up of three bodies or Sharira. These three bodies are: -

Sthula Sharira – Gross or Physical Body

Sukshma Sharira – Subtle or Astral Body.

Karana Sharira – Causal or Karmic Body.

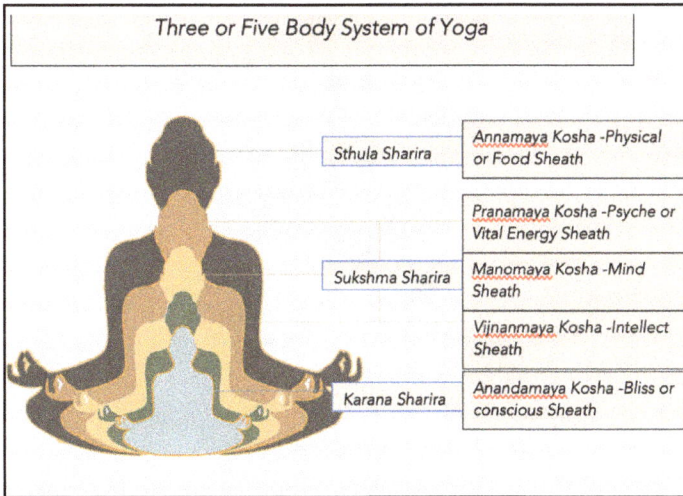

Within these three bodies are five sheaths (Pancha-Koshas), which are:-

- Annamaya Kosha – Food or Physical Body
- Pranamaya Kosha – Subtle Energy or Psychic Body
- Manomaya Kosha – Mind Body
- Vijnanamaya Kosha – Wisdom or Intellectual Body
- Anandamaya Kosha – Bliss or Spiritual Body.

Sthula Sharira or Physical Body

This is our physical or structural body including skin, bones, organs, muscles and everything that can be experienced by means of our senses.

Our physical body is made up of the Pancha-Mahabhutas or the five primary subtle elements. These five elements are: -

- Prathvi – solid or earth element
- Jala / Apas – liquid or water element
- Vayu – wind or air element
- Agni / Teja – fire or heat
- Akasha – ether, space or voidness

The Pancha-mahabhutas make up our body. According to Ashanga-Samgraha, predominance of Bhutas in our body constitution is as below:

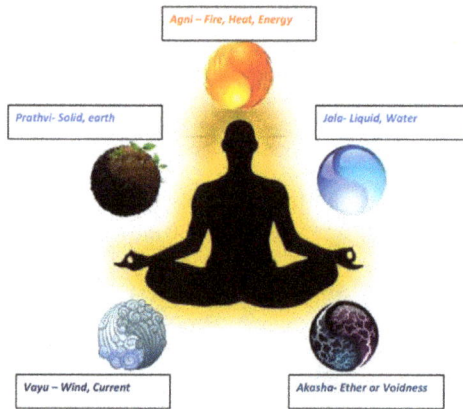

Body Constituent (Ayurveda)	Bhuta	Body Part
Rasa	Jala	plasma i.e. serum, white blood cells, lymphatic system
Rakta	Agni	red blood cells
Mamsa	Prithvi	muscle
Meda	Jala + Prithvi	fat
Asthi	Vayu	bones and cartilage
Majja	Jala	bone marrow, nerve tissue, connective tissue
Sukra	Jala	male/female reproductive organs

Sukshma Sharira or Astral Body

Our astral or subtle body is comprised of our mind and senses enabling us to experience pain and pleasure. It is the source of all our cognitive processes. In total there are 19 elements making up our astral body. These are:-

- Jnanendriyas – Five sense organs (sight, hearing, smell, touch, and taste)
- Karmendriyas – Five subtle organs of action; the feet (pada) movement, the hands (pani) grasp and hold, the rectum (payu) elimination, the genitals (upastha) procreate, and the mouth (vak) speaking
- Pancha Prana Vayus – Five subtle energy currents, which are prana, apana, samana, vyana and udana
- Four Atahakarana – Four inner subtle instruments, which are manas (the mind), buddhi (the intellect), chitta (the awareness) and ahamakara (the ego)

In the subtle body five cognitive senses receive all the information. The mind integrates this information and passes it down to buddhi or intellect for analysis as well as decision making. The mind also stores the information in the form of memories. Once a decision is made it is passed down to Karmendriyas for action and also stored in the mind as a memory. Our Anahmkara or sense of individuality plays a role to see things from our individual perspective and ego. When our Karmendriyas or instruments of actions are responding our ego makes us believe that I am doing it. The subtle body is also subject to changes and experience.

Karana Sharira or Causal Body

This is our seed body or blueprint of the gross and subtle bodies along with the life processes. This body cannot be experienced by means of our sense organs. Yoga guides us in a step by step manner to experience this Karmic Body and then liberate the soul from it in order to attain liberation. This body links us to our True Self or Atman. It contains all our previous experiences, memories, habits, and information of not only this life but all the previous lives we have lived. According to Upanishadic Wisdom, our causal and subtle bodies stay together and depart the physical body at the time of death and move on to the next body at the time of birth.

Pancha Koshas or The five sheaths

Annamaya kosha, the food or structural sheath: - This is our anatomical body or structure made of food. This sheath belongs to the Sthula Sharira.

Pranamaya kosha, the vital energy sheath: - This is the subtle energy body that transforms our anatomical body into the physiological or functional body. According to Upanishadic wisdom this body is composed of nadis, prana vayus, chakras, and Karmendriyas or organs of action.

Manomaya kosha, the mental sheath:- This is our mind body comprised of manas (mind), chitta (awareness or consciousness), jnanendriyas or sense organs. This transforms our anatomy and physiology in a living body which has the ability to feel and experience.

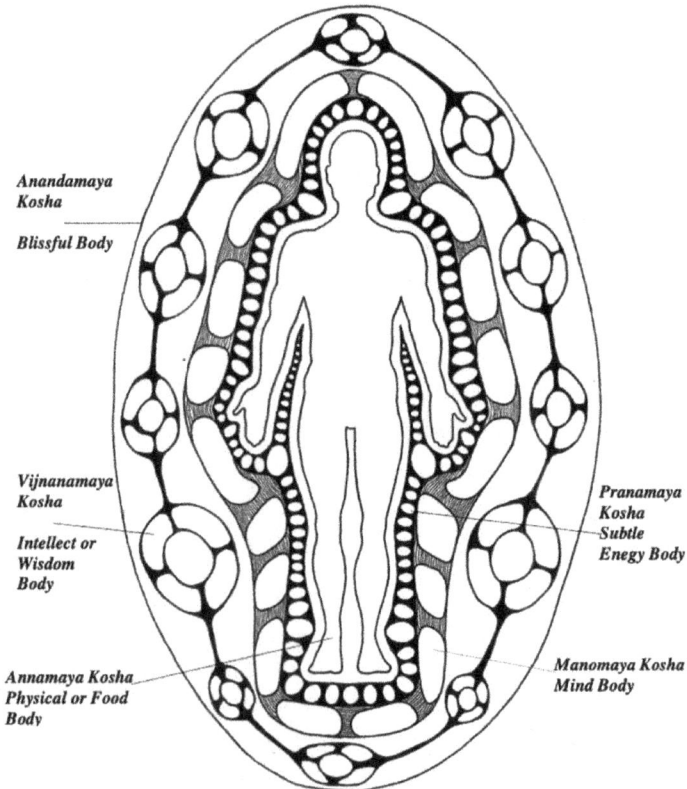

Pancha Kosha or Five Energy Bodies

Vijnanamaya kosha, the intellect or wisdom sheath: - This sheath is related with the astral body. It contains all the intellectual information (Buddhi) regarding our life processes, growth and evolution and has the ability to analyse the information we receive. It governs the ahamkara or ego and iccha-shakti or will-power. Our choices, discernment and descion-making abilities are manifestations of this Vijnanamaya Kosha.

Anandamaya kosha, the bliss sheath: - This is the all-pervading and central aspect of the causal body. This is the sheath relating to our Jiva or living being which experiences true wisdom, joy and bliss.

CHAPTER 3
by Yogachariya Jnandev Giri

Anatomy as per Ayurveda

Vedic teachings of ancient Ayurveda begins with the absolute concept of "atha pinde tat Brahmande, the individual jiva and body which represents the whole universe". This is developed further with "atha Brahmande tat Pinde", - "the universe represents the individual life." So the individual life and universe are interconnected and interrelated. The Prakriti or creations is constituted of Pancha-Mahabhutas and so is our body. According to Vedic teachings the Pancha-Mahabhutas and the Atma, Jiva or Soul together form the body. One of the Sanskrita verses mentions, "shat-dhatvatmak Purusha – gross existence of soul in the form of the body made of seven dhatus".

The Great Ayurveda master Charaka says:
Tatra shariram naam chetanadhishtanabhutam |
Panchmahabhutvikar samudayatmakam samyogavahi || Charaka Samhita 6. II
"Chetana (Consciousness) and the elements arising out of panchmahabhutas (five essential elements of earth, fire, water, air, space and ether) form the body".

The Samkhya and Upanishadic teachings on creation explain that the body is constituted of Panchamahabhutas. Each of these five elements bring forth the qualities and abilities of cognition by means of Jnanendriyas or sense organs as follows:-

Bhuta	Quality or characteristic and Indriya
Akasha – space or voidness	Sabda or sound, ear
Vayu – wind, air	Sparsha or touch, skin
Agni or Teja, fire, heat	Roop or form, view, eyes
Aapa, Jala or water	Rasa or taste, tongue
Prathvi, earth or solid	Gandha or smell, nose

It is understood that the Panchamahabhutas (earth, water, air, fire and ether) constitute the body, and through the Jnanendriyas or sense organs the Jiva perceives the qualities and characteristics of these elements. The nature of the Mahabhutas in terms of the organs of our body is as follows:

Prathvi Bhava (earthly or solid quality or nature)	Nails, bones, teeth, flesh, skin, excretion, beard, body hair, hair etc.
Jaliya Bhava (Liquid or watery nature or quality)	Fluids, kapha, pitta, urine, perspiration, and saliva.
Vayaviya Bhava (wind or air nature or quality)	Breathing, blinking and opening of the eyelids, speed, inspiration, dharana etc.
Agneya Bhava (fire or energy nature or quality)	Pitta, heat, the glow of the body, view, eyesight etc
Akashiya Bhav (Nature and quality of ether or voidness)	All holes, hollow places, small and big strotra, vocal system and ear system

Ayurveda states that "shiryate tat shariram", which means "that which degenerates is known as the body". Our body is a gradual accumulation of panchamahabhutas as part of our growth as well as also gradually decomposing or degrading as we move through old age, disease and death. In this process the panchamahabhutas return to their source.

This process of creation and decomposition of the body carries on continuously.

We pick the elements from the surrounding environment knowingly or unknowingly via the body and assimilate them. This gives rise to desires, hunger, and thirst. Also due to access, to lack of dependence and toxicity of these subtle elements we also experience liking and disliking, or attraction and repulsion, towards these elements. If you reflect on your own life and how we develop attraction or aversion towards food, drink, cold, heat, water, etc it is really a sign of access to or lack of a particular element or toxicity in your body.

According to the Ayurvedic text Sushruti all the natural processes in our body may result in one of the three: Visarga, Aadan or Vikshepa.
Visargadanvikshepe somsuryanila yatha |
Dharyanti jagddeham kaphapitta nilastatatha || Sushrut ||

Visarg a (giving strength, Aadan (taking away of strength), Vikshepa (distraction or disturbance). Behind these three outcomes, there are three strengths in nature: Chandra, Surya and Vayu (moon, sun and wind). Within the body these outcomes are governed or performed by Kapha, Pitta and Vata.

These three principles or Doshas (Vata, Pitta and Kapha) are governing the integration and disintegration of the constituents in the body. Charak Samhita describes Tridoshas as follows:-

Kapha is a white coloured substance, which is cold, heavy, slow, sticky and glossy. Even if it is subtle or gross, it has these qualities. As per Ayurveda, kapha amounts to six palms full. That means it can be in liquid form too. Even if the oily part of the kapha is demonstrated through the organs, its other characteristics are according to its functions.

Pitta is hot, sharp, expansive in nature with a particular or strong smell. Even if these are demonstrated through organs, other characteristics are as per their functios. Pitta is five palmfuls. This also is a liquid substance.
Vata is dry and less cold when compared with kapha, tiny and movable.

This substance is of a mobile nature and not related to body organs. It is called as "Avyaktovyaktakarma", which means "although it is not expressed on its own, it is expressed through actions".

Further, Ayurveda explains that the health or illness of the body depends on the balance or imbalance of the tri-doshas. Our bodily functions and our movements are dependent on these principles too. Even though the Pancha-Mahabhutas are constitutional elements of body formation, primarily the three elements (aap – liquid, teja – energy and vayu - wind) are the main elements of our functions. These elements seek the help of Prathvi and Akasha elements to carry out their functions.

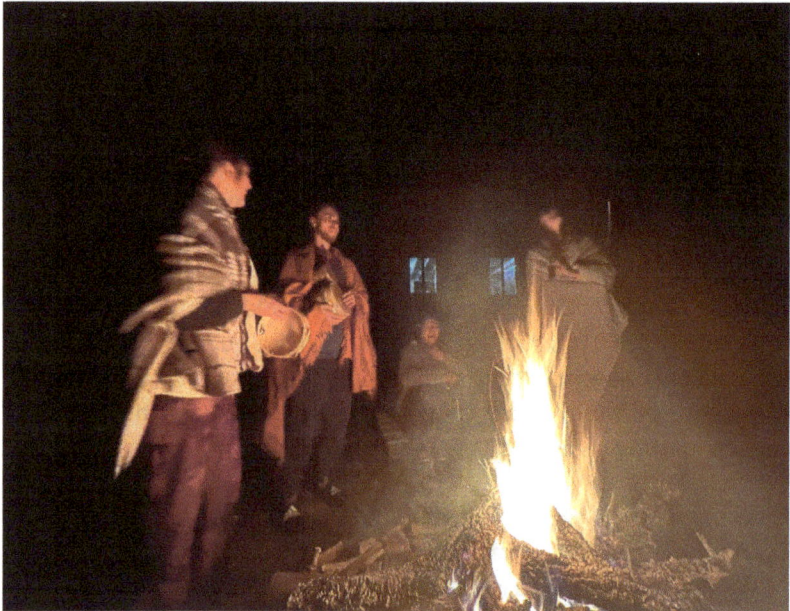

CHAPTER 4
Tri-dosha: Three Doshas
(Vata, Pitta, Kapha)

by Yogachariya Jnandev Giri

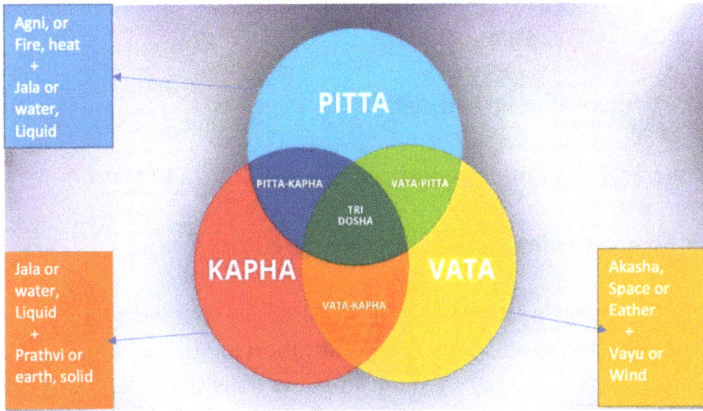

Agni, or Fire, heat + Jala or water, Liquid

Jala or water, Liquid + Prathvi or earth, solid

Akasha, Space or Eather + Vayu or Wind

PITTA

PITTA-KAPHA

VATA-PITTA

TRI DOSHA

KAPHA

VATA

VATA-KAPHA

The Ancient Ayurveda, science of herbal remedies, yoga therapy and naturopathy, is the oldest known form of healthcare in the world. It comes from the Vedic culture of Bharat-Varsh (known as India in a modern context). It is commonly believed to have arrived through the sincere effort of great Rishis, Sages and Therapists in India around 5000 or more years ago.

In Recent decades, Ayurveda has become more popular and has been adapted according to modern scientific research studies. Swami Ramdev's Yoga and Ayurveda Movement has now made Ayurveda available to a wider community in India. Ayurveda offers us the potential to heal chronic diseases, cleanse our body-mind system and improve our health and longevity.

Maharishi Patanjali offers us three healing aspects :–
- Ayurveda – for purifying our body for health and evolution
- Vyakarana or grammar – for purifying our language
- Yoga Darshan – for purifying our mind and attaining self-realisation.

Ayurveda is a science of understanding our wholisitic self and offers us many key concepts as follows :-

Sapta Dhatus – Seven constitutional aspects

Tri-Doshas – Vata, Pitta, Kapha

Tri-Gunas – Sattva, Rajas, Tamas

Ahara – Vihra or lifestyle and diet

Samaskaras and Karma – Genetic, Epigenetic, Birth, and Mind

Pranic Energy – Prana Vayus or vital energy currents.

Ayurvedic Science provides scientific tools to understand our Individual self from gross to subtle, from our constitution to our own unique nature. This also explains the way we think and interact with other people. This enables us to understand our choices, cravings and desires, which can help us make better or healthier choices bringing holistic transformation into our lives.

Ayurveda explains that, "disease is the natural result of living out of harmony with one's constitution". Our constitution is the inherited balance of energies within our body, mind and pranic energy system. This describes our true nature at the most fundamental level. This unique constitutional science of Doshas determines everything from our physical structure of bones, muscles, tissues etc to our predisposition toward various health threats. It also defines what we are naturally attracted to and what we repel. It further details what helps in establishing and maintaining our nature and inherited qualities and what will cause imbalance and result in disease or sickness. Because we are different in terms of our constitutional energy, the path of optimum health and wellbeing will be different for each individual.

This Ayurvedic Science of understanding our true nature and energy constitution is known as the Science of Tridoshas. Tri-Doshas are defined as the three fundamental energy principles which govern the function of our bodies on a physical, mental, emotional and intellectual level. These three energy principles are known as Vata, Pitta, and Kapha. Each individual has a unique balance of these three energies. Many of us will be dominant in one of the three, or a mixture of two or more.

On the most fundamental level, pitta is our metabolism, kapha is our structure, and vata is the mobility that brings action and life into creation. Without all three energies, we simply could not exist.

To determine a person's constitution, a Clinical Ayurvedic consultation with an Ayurveda specialist is necessary. This physical, emotional, and spiritual evaluation identifies the balance of energies in a person's body as well as areas of imbalance. Once the nature of the person and the imbalance identified, we can design a yoga therapy plan according to our 12 point model which includes diet, lifestyle, hatha yoga, pranayama, relaxation techniques, yogic attitude, contemplations etc, in order to restore and maintain balance.

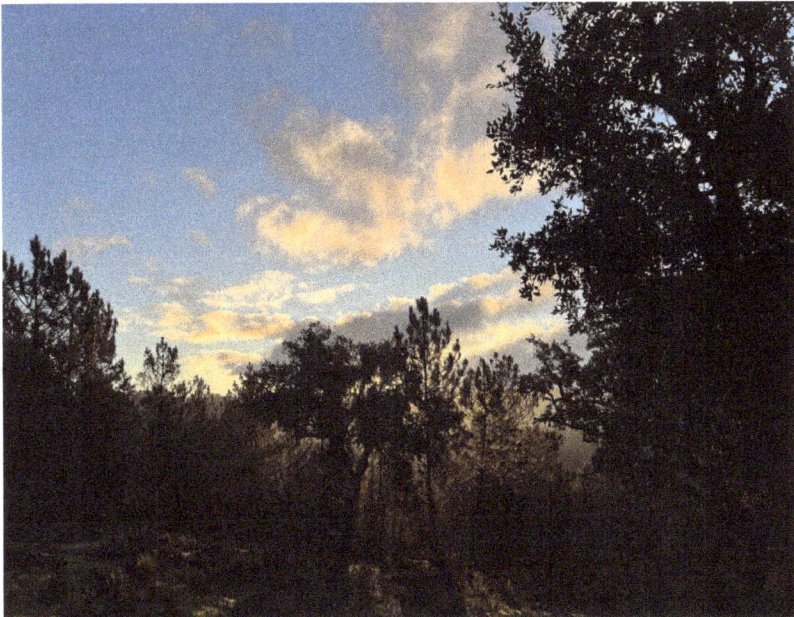

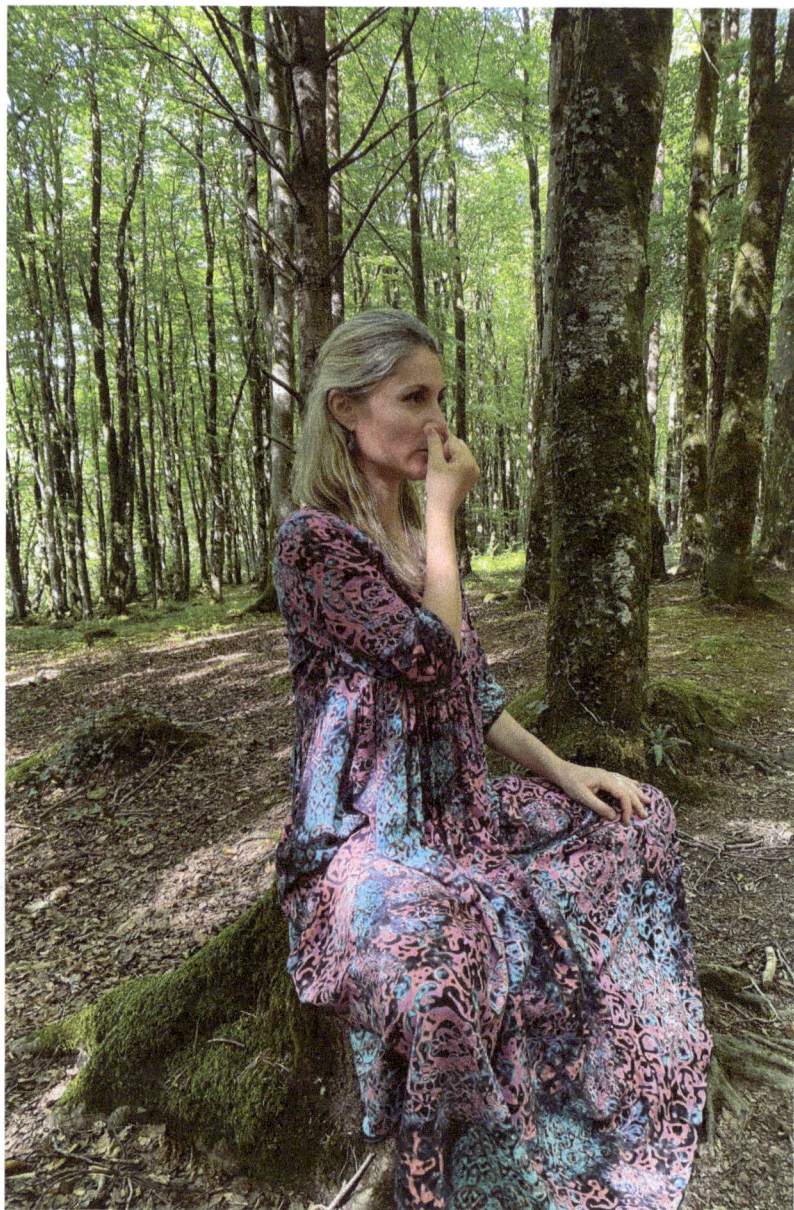

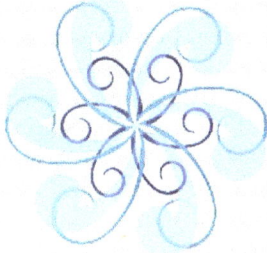

The Vata Dosha

Vata Dosha is known to be made of the wind (Vayu) and the ether or space (Akasha) elements. Vata Dosha contains similar qualities to Vayu and Akasha Bhutas. Vata has similar qualities to the wind – light, cool, dry and mobile. People with Vata qualities experience these qualities. Their bodies are often light, bones are thin and they have dry skin and hair. They tend to move and talk quickly. When people with Vata quality are out of harmony they may lose weight, suffer with constipation and a weak immunity and nervous system.

Those with Vata quality tend to be talkative, enthusiastic, creative, flexible and energetic in their personality. When they are out of balance they may easily become confused and overwhelmed, find it difficult to focus and make decisions and also suffer with sleep disorders. Stress is a strong triggering point for people with Vata quality. Emotionally they suffer with worry, fear and anxiety.

Common Health Issues Associated with Vata :- anxiety, constipation, insomnia, arthritis, chronic pain or Parkinson's disease

To establish balance to Vata quality, we need a program emphasising the opposing qualities of warmth, heaviness, nourishment, moistness and stability.

Diet – cooked grains like rice and lentils, cooked vegetables and intake of warm milk and spices.

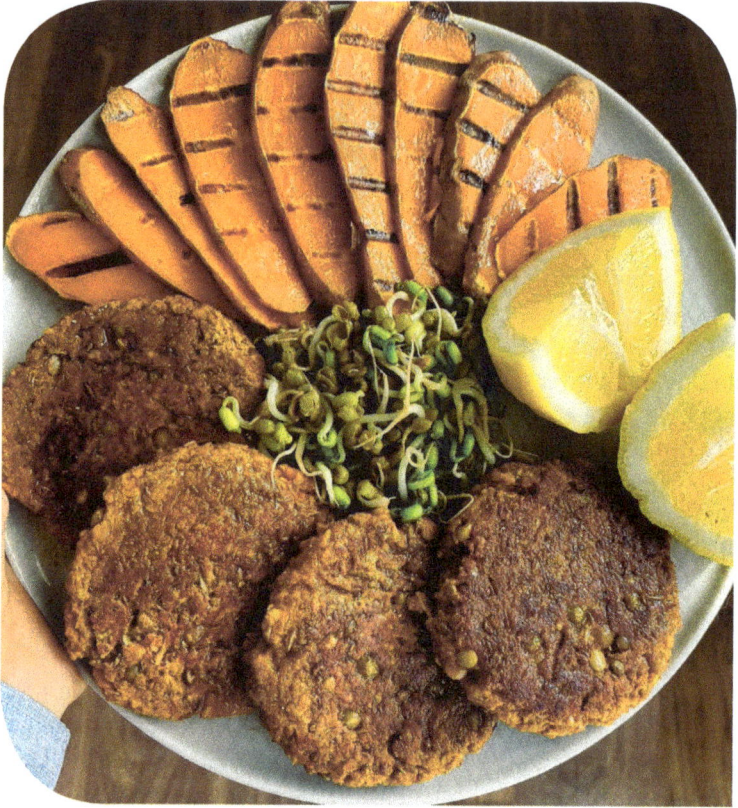

Fruits - Sweet fruits such as bananas, coconuts, apples, figs, grapefruits, grapes, mangos, melons, oranges, papayas, peaches, pineapples, plums, berries, cherries, apricots and avocados.

Dried fruits can also be eaten, but not too much. The following general rule applies to fruit consumption: at least one hour before or after meals, but not in the evening.

Vegetables:- Cooked: asparagus, red beets, carrots, sweet potatoes, radish, zucchini, spinach (in small quantities), sprouts (in small quantities), tomatoes (in small quantities), celery, garlic, and onions (only steamed).

Herbs – Pungent herbs like oregano, rosemary and sage and all the kitchen spices like ginger, coriander, cumin or cayenne are recommended to increase the digestive fires and for stimulating, warming, drying and dispersing.

Ayurvedic programs also include colour and aroma therapies, detoxification, yoga, and meditation.

Hatha Yoga recommendations for Vata Balance:- Asanas engaging the lower body (lower back, hips and legs) with holding them gently (Isometric) like Vriksha-Asana, Meru-Asana, Veera-Asana Variations, Veera-Bhadra-Asana Series can help us through grounding our feet and stabilising our energies. All variations of the Pawan-Mukta Kriyas are some of the best kriyas to release any trapped wind and balance the Vata quality.

Pranayama for Vata Balance:- Anuloma-Viloma, Nadi Sodhana and Savitri Pranayama.

Mudra – Prathvi Mudra. For Prathvi Mudra join the tip of ring finger and thumb while keeping the other three fingers straight.

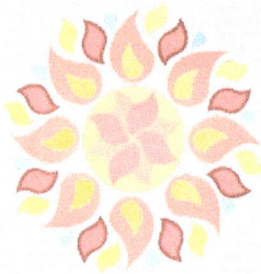

The Pitta Dosha

The Pitta Dosha is constituted from Agni (fire or energy) and Jala (water or liquid) where fire is more predominant. People with Pitta quality tend to have qualities of fire :- hot, sharp and penetrating. This is also volatile and oily due to the water element. People with Pitta quality tend to feel warm with oily skin, penetrating eyes and sharp features. These people tend to have moderate weight and a good physique.

When out of balance, Pitta dominating people suffer with diarrhoea, infections, skin rashes and problems related to the liver, spleen and blood.

Pitta personalities tend to be highly focused, competitive, courageous, energetic, and clear in communication. These people in life tend to excel at solving problems and thrive under the stress. They can also be intense and speak very sharply. They are good at making friends and fear making enemies. Emotionally Pitta people are challenged by the heated emotions of anger, resentment and jealousy.

Further Pitta quality people can be well-structured, good in managing projects and concentrate very well. They can be good teachers and their lessons are logically organised, which make them easy to follow. The Pitta types tend to spend money more systematically and prudently.

To bring balance to Pitta qualities, we need to design a program emphasising the opposing qualities of coolness, heaviness and dryness.

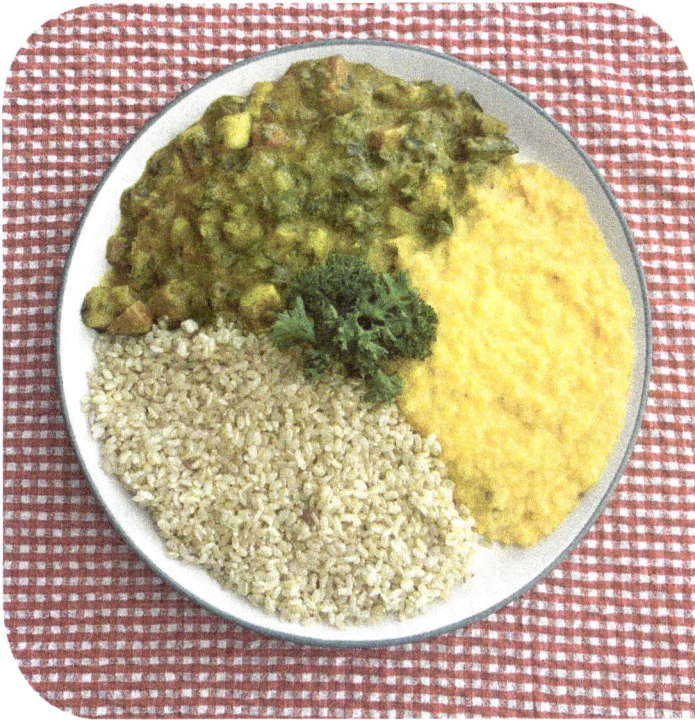

Diet :- The Pitta types can be soothed by a predominantly vegetarian diet, bitter vegetables are recommended. The food should not be too spicy, salty, or sour and it is recommended to eat cool food in summer and hot food in winter.

Fruits :- Sweet fruits like: apples, avocados, coconuts, figs, melons, oranges, pears, plums, pomegranates, and mangos are recommended to balance Pitta quality. Avoid dried fruits.

Vegetables :- Sweet and bitter: asparagus, cabbage, cucumber, cauliflower, celery, green beans, lettuce, peas, parsley, potatoes, zucchini, sprouts, cress, chicory, and mushrooms.

Grains :- Barley, oats (cooked), basmati or white rice, and wheat.

Spices :- cilantro, cinnamon, turmeric, cardamom, fennel, and some black pepper.

Milk Products : Butter (unsalted), ghee, goats milk, cows milk, pans, and cheese. Soy milk and tofu as a vegan substitute.

A Clinical Ayurvedic program may also include aromas, colours, massage, detoxification, yoga, and meditation.

Hatha Yoga for Pitta Dosha :- The seat of Pitta is our stomach and digestive area. Backbends and twists are highly recommended hatha yoga practices for balancing Pitta. Dhanurasana, Ustrasana, Chakrasana, Ardha Matsendrasana and Brahma Danda Asana Series are some of the typical Asanas for Pitta quality. A gentle, effortless, conscious and mindful flow or Kriya Yoga to rejuvenate, relax, develop patience, calmness and become receptive.

Pranayama for Pitta :- Shitali, Shitakari and Kaki Pranayama.

Mudra for Pitta :- Prana Mudra.

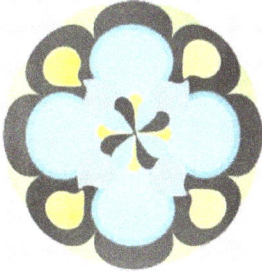

- Elements – Jala and Prathvi
- Qualities- cool, moist, stable and heavy
- Body- dense, heavy bones, lustrous, supple skin, low metabolism with large stocky physique
- Personality – heaviness, stable nature, resilience to quick fluctuations.
- Issues – depression, obesity, lethargy and diabetes

The Kapha Dosha

Kapha Dosha is constituted of Jala (water or liquid) and Prathivi (earth or solid) elements predominantly. Kapha is cool, moist, stable and heavy in quality. In our body these qualities manifest as dense, heavy bones, lustrous and supple skin, low metabolism, and large stocky frames. People with kapha quality tend to feel cold.

People with Kapha quality like regularity and routine in their life, which is something natural in them. They also have a tendency towards overeating, avoiding exercise and sleeping excessively.

Kapha people also tend to hold onto things, money, and people. This coupled with water retention makes life difficult for them in terms of relationships, but financially helps them gain wealth and possessions.

When Kapha people are out of balance they are prone to weight gain and health problems associated with respiration and sinuses due to accumulation of mucous. People with Kapha quality are also prone to non-insulin dependent diabetes mellitus.

The Kapha quality can be also seen in our personality in terms of heaviness, a stable nature and stable personality, showing resilience to sudden fluctuations. People with a Kapha nature are able to deal with stress efficiently and with ease.

When out of balance, they don't like change as by nature they are comfort seekers, which can lead to a lack of motivation and general feelings of becoming stuck in life. When Kapha is out of balance, people suffer with the heavy emotions of depression, obesity and lethargy.

To bring balance to a Kapha personality, we need to offer a program with the opposing qualities of lightness, dryness and warmth.

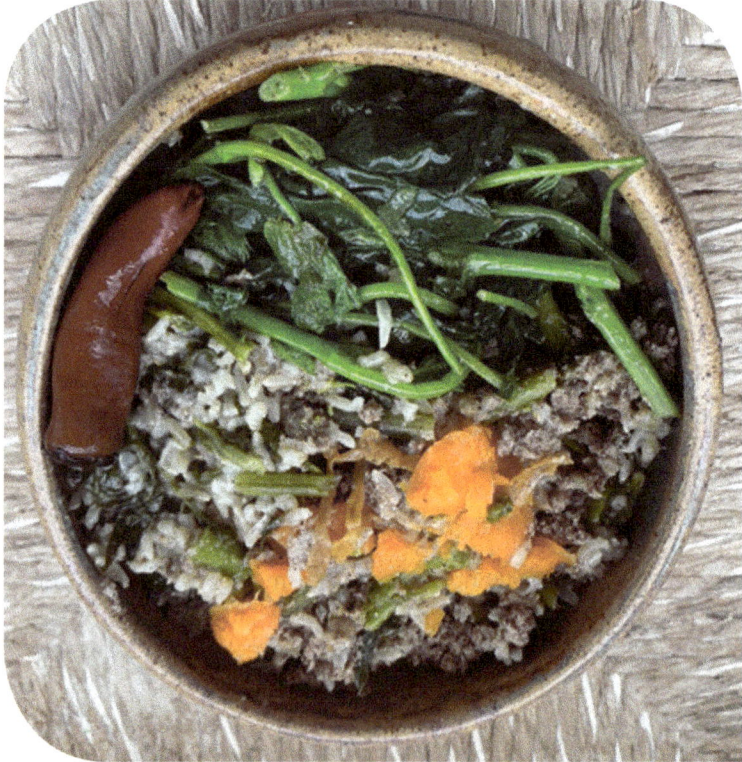

Diet :- "Eat less than you feel hungry for or are craving. Good foods are spicy or well-seasoned, dry, and antioedema."

Fruits :- Apple, berries, cherries, mangos, peaches, pears, and raisins are recommended. Dried fruits other than figs and plums should be avoided.

Vegetables :- Spicy and bitter, red beets, cabbage, carrots, cauliflower, celery, eggplant, garlic, lettuce, mushrooms, onions, parsley, peas, radish, spinach, sprouts, fennel, and brussels sprouts.

Grains :- Barley, corn, millet, oats, basmati rice (small quantities).

Spices – All spices especially pungent herbs like cloves, guggul, ginger, turmeric.

Milk and Milk Products :- Reduced-fat milk in small quantities avoid fatty cheeses and curd (quark). Vegan milk options are preferable in general.

Hatha Yoga :- The seat of Kapha is our upper digestive tract and chest area. Dynamic Practices like Vinyasa, Surya Namaskars, stronger yoga poses can help detoxifying ama or toxic build-up and boost metabolism. They need to feel full energy, lightness, letting go and forgiveness, clarity and illumination through the yoga practice.

Pranayama :- Bhastrika and Anunasika Pranayama.

Kapha Nasaka Mudra :- This mudra is performed by placing the ring and the little fingers on the base of the thumb and then bringing gentle pressure of the thumb upon these fingers. Keep the other two fingers straight.
Effects: This mudra increases the Pitta quality and decreases the Kapha quality.

Samaan Mudra – can be used to balance three Doshas.

CHAPTER 5

SKB
Activated *Vegan Food* ®

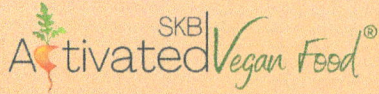

AYURVEDA DOSHA TEST

Check the box next to the quality that resembles your physical characteristics/behaviour the most. Then add up the ticks in each column.

PHYSICAL CHARACTERISTICS	VATA/AIR	√	PITTA/BILE	√	KAPHA/MUCUS	√
WALKING PACE	Fast, irregular, you go where the wind blows		Brisk, purposeful		Slow, graceful	
STRUCTURAL ABNORMALITIES	Nasal septum defects, Bowlegs, bone spurs		Few		Lumps, cysts	
EYES	Active, dry, unsteady		Penetrating gaze, red or yellow sclera		Prominent, oily, white sclera	
WEIGHT GAIN	Hard to gain weight		Maintain steady weight		Easily gain weight	
LOCATION OF WEIGHT	Around waist		Evenly deposited		Below waist	
FOOD INTAKE	Variable		High amount at one time		Steady	
BOWEL HABITS	Irregular, not every day		Twice or more per day		Regular, every day	
PERSPIRATION	Hardly ever		More than average		Little, greasy	
DIGESTION	Easily upset		Can eat anything		Slow, feelings of fullness	
FOOD CRAVING	Erratic - no desire or sudden strong craving		Very strong, do not like to skip meals		Low, easily skip meals	
	TOTAL		TOTAL		TOTAL	

BEHAVIOR CHARACTERISTICS	VATA/AIR	√	PITTA/BILE	√	KAPHA/MUCUS	√
TASK PERFORMANCE	Quickly, with enthusiasm		Intensively		Methodically	
ATTENTION SPAN	Short		Medium, intense, then move on		Long	
LIFE INTERESTS	Many, always something new, drop after newness wears off		Many, intense, obsessions		Few, deep, gives up when it needs too much work.	
REACTION TO A PROBLEM	Worried		Irritated, angry		Calm, stable	
APPROACH NEW INFORMATION	Quick grasp of new and exotic		Quickly digest information		Review material thoroughly	
SEX DRIVE	High, erratic, kinky		Moderate		Steady	
SPEECH	Quick, chaotic, continuous		Convincing, direct, sharp		Slow, quiet, definite	
RESPONSE TO THREAT	Very readily		Fairly easily		Not easily	
FOOD PREFERENCES	Sweets, salads, fruit		Spicy, fried		Greasy, salty	
FALLING ASLEEP	Stay up late Hard to fall asleep		Stay up if involved and stimulated Easy to get up early		Early, easily	
	TOTAL		TOTAL		TOTAL	

Now add up the physical and behavioural characteristics:

	TOTAL		TOTAL		TOTAL	

If you have more than 10 total points in one of the three rows (*vata, pitta or kapha*) then work on balancing your dominant dosha using the following table:

BALANCING YOUR CONSTITUTION (DOSHA)

	Vata – air	Pitta – bile	Kapha – mucus
QUALITIES	MOVEMENT *(Air and Ether)* Cold, light, dry, unsteady, undisciplined, hyperactive, quick, changeable.	TRANSFORMATION *(Fire and Water)* Hot, intense, strong, extreme, sharp, caustic.	PROTECTION *(Earth and Water)* Heavy, slow, persistent, stable, concentrated, soft, greasy.
HABITS/QUALITIES TO ENCOURAGE	Routine, discipline, meditation.	Relaxation, silence, modesty.	Movement, change.
TASTES FOR BALANCE	Salty Sour *(lemon)* Sweet *(carrot)*	Sweet *(fig)*, Bitter *(raw greens)* Astringent *(chickpeas)*	Bitter *(kale)* Spicy *(hot pepper)* Astringent *(lentils)*
TASTES TO AVOID	Bitter, astringent, very spicy	Pungent, sour *(cheese, tomatoes)*, salty	Sweet, salty, sour
FOOD FOR BALANCE	Sprouted pulses with digestive formula, mung dal, green peas. Vegetables: prefer cooked with digestive formula and oil added in the end: cooked beets, carrots, asparagus, sweet potatoes, peas, broccoli, celery, zucchini, green beans. Spices: *(gradually increase to maximum 1 tablespoon per meal)* black pepper, mustard seed, cumin, ginger, cinnamon, cardamom. Rice, wheat, and all nuts (*soaked in water*). Oranges, bananas, avocado, grapes, peaches, melons, fresh figs, soaked dates, mangoes, sweet pineapple, apples (*cooked*). Non vegan: All dairy (*warm, not cold*) and eggs.	Lentils, Mung beans, tofu. Olive oil, coconut oil. Asparagus, cabbage, cucumber, carrots, broccoli, cauliflower, sprouts, celery, and green leafy vegetables. Barley, oats, white rice, wheat. Grapes, coconut, cherries, avocado, melons, mangoes, pomegranates, sweet oranges, plums, pineapples. Sunflower seeds, pumpkin seeds. Non vegan: milk, butter, and ghee.	Beans, raw greens, almost all vegetables *(preferably raw, without oil and salt)* Barley, rye, corn, millet. Hot spices. Pears, apples, raisins, pomegranates, honey, Turmeric, ginger.
FOOD TO AVOID	Dry, raw, light, cold, complicated.	Dry, light, hot, oily.	Oily, cold, heavy.

CHAPTER 6

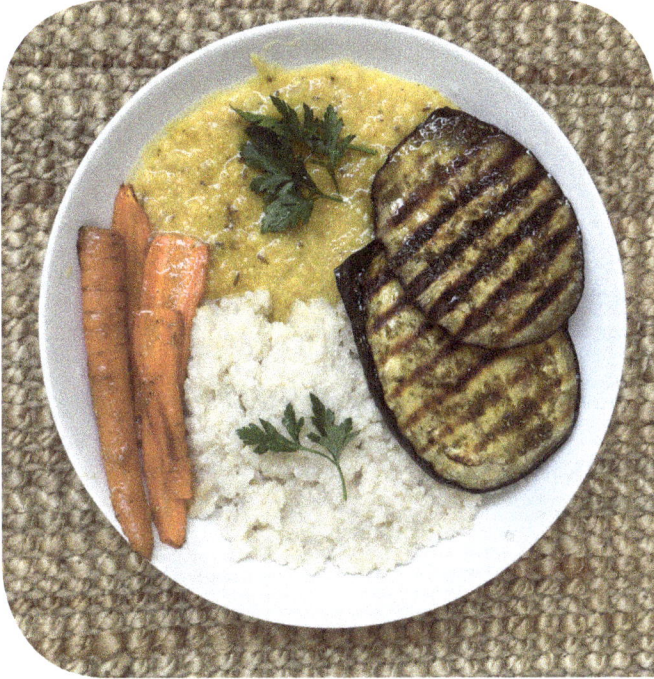

Yogic diet
Ayurveda Simplified

Guna/dosha/rasa theory
By Yogacharini Anandhi – Korina Kontaxaki

Ayurveda is a treatment system based on ancient Indian texts and teachings. With connections to the Yogic and Hindu way of life, it appears that Yoga, Hinduism and Ayurveda are interrelated and were practiced together, as they complement each other.

Ayurveda induces a way of life and a dietary system that will maintain physical strength, health and vitality. The healthy body can then aid mental concentration and clarity, which will also assist in meditation practice.

The theory of Ayurveda is vast, but we will focus on 3 key elements, which will help us understand how food can become both a cure and a tool for mental clarity.

1.   Guna – Quality
2.   Dosha – Constitution
3.   Shadrasa – The 6 Flavors

GUNA – Quality

Life, as we experience it in its material form, is in constant motion. It exists and changes between 3 qualities/Guna:

1. Excitable – Rajas Guna – Intense quality, without limits
2. Dull – Tamas Guna – Slow, heavy quality, with obstacles
3. Purified – Sattva Guna – Ideal quality, always acting at the right time and place

All actions, thoughts, emotions, and habits, move between these 3 qualities.

When our life is excitable (rajasic) or dull (tamasic), it is separate from the truth and the source of energy that nourishes the entire universe. The purified quality (sattvic), is the one that has a balanced flow of energy between the 2 opposites of Rajas and Tamas, and moves at the centre of all, so it is in tune with the true nature of someone who is connected with the Source.

(*The word Sattva comes from the words Sat - truth + Tvam - to be, and translates as "True Being")

Each of us can be intense, passive, or balanced, depending on the circumstances. However, various habits may encourage or reduce these qualities. One of these habits is the food we eat.

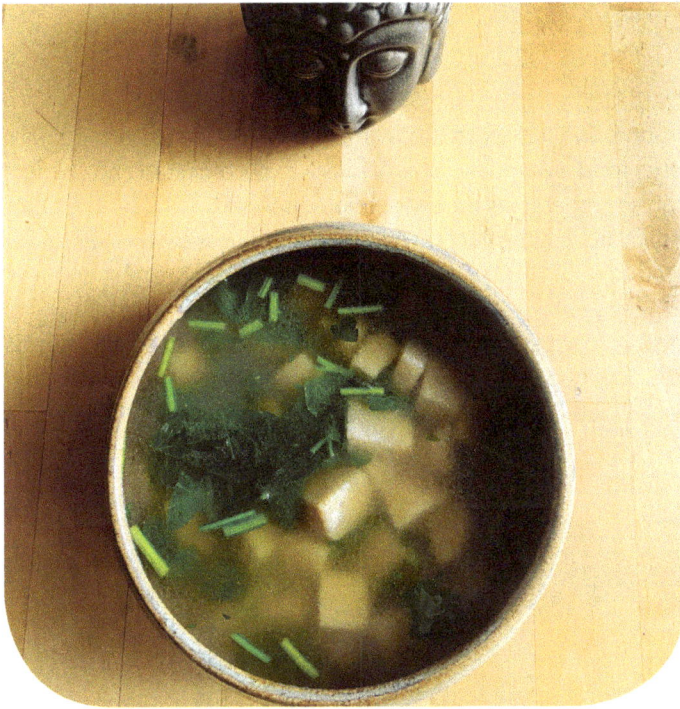

We can therefore divide food into:

1. Aggressive (Rajasic)
2. Passive (Tamasic)
3. Balanced (Sattvic)

If we eat Sattvic food, we encourage physical and mental purification and balance.

Examples of food types

1. Aggressive Food - caffeine, chocolate, high spice content, high salt content.
2. Passive Food - fish, pasteurized dairy, non-fresh, processed, overcooked, pre-cooked and re-heated.
3. Balanced Food - plant-based food, natural, raw or freshly cooked, seasonal.

Garlic and Onion: While these foods have
both Rajasic and Tamasic qualities, the end result is Tamasic.

Meat and eggs: Digestion requires high energy demands, so their consumption results in lethargy in a person (Tamas)

Mushrooms and fermented vegetables: It is said that they are passive (Tamasic) food. But mushrooms are very easily digested and fermented vegetables (vegetables that have been through natural fermentation) aid and improve digestion, thus reducing the possibility of inertia. Eat in moderation.

In conclusion, a diet that is "alive" with natural, unprocessed plant-based food is a very good way of keeping the physical/mental/spiritual system in balance (Sattva), united with the true source of energy (Prana).

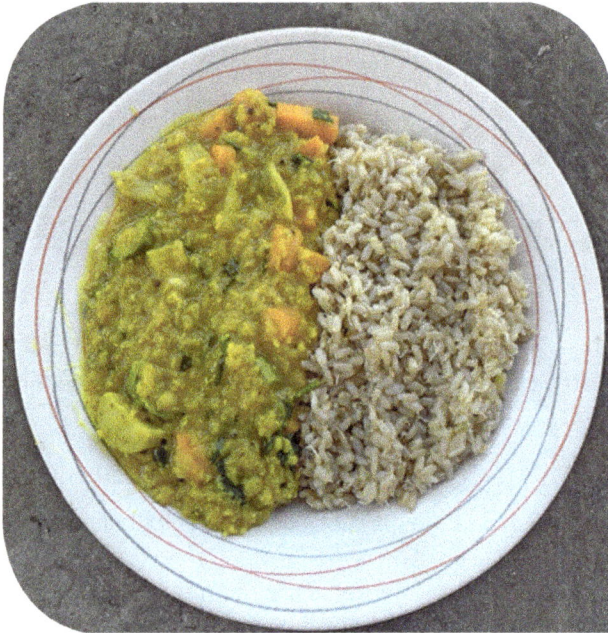

Shadrasa – The 6 Flavors

According to Ayurveda, in order to have a complete sense of fullness and satisfaction, every meal must contain all 6 flavors. In this way we can ensure that we are including all the elements; water, fire, earth, air, and ether in our meal.

The 6 Flavors
1.   Sweet (water and earth)
2.   Sour (water and fire)
3.   Pungent (air and fire)
4.   Bitter (air and ether)
5.   Salty (earth and fire)
6.   Astringent (air and earth)

*Note that the ether element that cleanses the blood and the energy in the body, can only be found in bitter flavors.

Sources of the Flavors
1. Sweet: Grains, pasta, rice, bread, starchy vegetables, sugar, honey, molasses
2. Sour: Citrus fruits, berries, tomatoes, pickled foods
3. Salty: Table salt, soy sauce
4. Pungent: Peppers, chilies, onions, garlic, cayenne, black pepper, cloves, ginger, mustard
5. Bitter: Leafy greens, green and yellow vegetables, kale, celery, broccoli, sprouts, beets
6. Astringent: Lentils, dried beans, green apples, grape skins, cauliflower, pomegranates, tea

No single flavor should dominate in any food. Avoid food being too sweet, too spicy, too salty, too sour, or too bitter.

When cooking, make sure you add a touch of all the flavors to your meal. In this way, you may gradually come to the surprising conclusion that you no longer crave a sweet dessert!

Adding spices and herbs to our food is essential for balancing out the flavor.

Dosha – Constitution

In order to function properly, the human system of body, mind and emotions, produces 3 substances:

1. Kapha - Mucus, for protection
2. Pitta - Bile, for transformation (breaking down)
3. Vata - Air, for movement

The nature of these Dosha is not only related to the body; there are also mental and emotional effects. For example, if a person experiences fear, the body can produce mucus for protection. Since the body/mind/emotions complex is interdependent, whatever happens on one level, is transferred to the other levels. This is the reason why we focus so much on the idea of how a proper diet will inevitably affect the mind as well.

Personal Constitution (Dosha)

According to Ayurveda, every person is born with a specific constitution, which produces the 3 Dosha in a specific way. So, under certain circumstances, some people may produce more mucus, bile or air than what is considered 'normal' levels. If one of the Dosha is regularly produced in excess, it creates problems for the system (the body/mind/emotion complex)

- Excessive mucus creates lethargy, the inability to take quick action, slow reaction to situations, slow metabolism, and lung problems.

- Excessive bile creates nervousness, despair, anger, impatience, stomach ulcers, and skin problems.

- Excessive air creates mental instability, fear, neurological problems, joint pain, bad digestion and absorption, intense energy followed by low energy, drowsiness, and bloating.

Our daily food intake directly affects the mucus/bile/air secretion in the body, so it is advisable to avoid the foods that are burdening your system. Take the Dosha test attached, to discover if you have a Dosha imbalance.

In conclusion, our aim should be to add 'alive' Sattvic food, according to our constitution (Dosha), and to ensure that we are including all 6 flavor (Shadrasa) in our daily food intake or at least in our main meal.

By following the Ayurvedic theory on quality, constitution, and the 6 flavours we can:
- Improve our psychology, vitality, and immune system.
- Reduce various tendencies we have for certain illnesses, or even weaken mental/psychological habits that are rather more harmful than useful.

This text is part of the Activated Vegan Food Seminar® by Anandhi Korina Kontaxaki . You can find the full AVF guide here: https://yogalifewithanandhi.com/

CHAPTER 7

Dosha And Their Guna + Rasa

by Yogacharini Anandhi – Korina Kointaxaki

In Ayurveda we work not only with the Dosha but with the Gunas (qualities) of each dosha, for better results. This is because we might have imbalances in different qualities which represent different Doshas. When we work on a constitution, we try with different questions to understand which Gunas (qualities) the care seeker has, and give them practices that increase the opposite guna.

Here are the 10 main gunas and their opposites
Here are the dosha with their gunas/tastes/elements and some spices to balance their qualities.

Guna	Opposite guna
Guru Heavy (K)	Laghu Light (VP)
Manda Slow/dull (K)	Tikshna Sharp (VP)
Sīta Cold (VK)	Uṣṇa Hot (P)
Ślakṣṇa Smooth/slimy (PK)	Khara Rough (V)
Drava Liquid (PK)	Sāndra Solid/dense (K)
Mrda Soft (PK)	Kaṭhina Hard (VK)
Sthira Static (K)	Cala Mobile (VP)
Sthūla Big/Gross (K)	Sūkṣma Subtle (VP)
Picchila Cloudy/sticky (K)	Viśadā Clear (VP)
Snigdha Oily (KP)	Ruksha dry (V)

Dosha	VATA	PITTA	KAPHA
Element taste	Ether+ air (bitter)	Fire + water (salty)	Earth + water (sweet)
Minor tastes	Pungent (air+ fire) and astringent (air+ earth)	Pungent (air + fire) and sour (fire+ earth)	Salty (fire+ water) and astringent (air+ earth)
Spices	Anise **Ginger** Cardamom Oregano **Cinnamon** **Lemon** Nutmeg	**Coriander** Cumin Turmeric **Lime** Mint **Parsley** Liquorice	Basil Chilli Cloves **Ginger** Garlic Turmeric **Mint** Nutmeg **Pepper** Rosemary Sage Mustard
Guna	Dry Light Cold Rough Subtle Mobile Clear	Oily Sharp Hot Light Mobile Liquid	Heavy Slow/dull Cold Oily Slimy/smooth Dense Soft Static Sticky Gross

Dosha and their gunas in detail with some foods to balance with the opposite guna

PITTA GUNA (fire and water)	OPPOSITE GUNA
Oily (oily hair, oily face, loose stools, acne) Fried food Too much oil Roasted nuts	**Dry** (bitter and astringent) Greens Sprouted pulses (Barley, buckwheat, corn dry fruit and vegetables.)
Sharp (very strong digestion, ulcer, irritability, anger) Hot peppers Alcohol Fermented food Sour food Coffee	**Slow/dull** (astringent and sweet) Aloe Rose Wheat
Hot (rashes, skin irritation, anger, stress) Pungent Garlic Honey	**Cold** (bitter, astringent, sweet) Apples Coconut Cucumber
Light (white hair, photosensitivity, light nervous system) Boiled or steamed vegetables	**Heavy** (sweet and astringent) Nuts Avocado Dates bananas
Mobile (hyperactivity, impatience) Eating on the go Eating while watching tv	**Static** Eating as a ceremony Eating slowly
Liquid (thin blood, bleeding) Juices Milk	**Solid** Fruit Rice

VATA GUNA (air and ether)	OPPOSITE GUNA
Dry (dry skin, dry stools, constipation, fear, pain) Dry fruit, Crackers Pop corn	**Oily** (sweet) Nuts Oil Fried food
Light (underweight, unable to focus) Raw food, Vegetables Boiled or steamed food	**Heavy** (sweet, salty) Wheat Meat Eggs
Cold (cold feet and hands, bad circulation) Raw food Leftovers Frozen	**Hot** (sour, pungent) Black pepper White cheese
Rough (rough skin and hair) Beans Raw vegetables Apples	**Smooth/slimy** Dhal Cheese Oil Cooked apples
Subtle (unable to make decisions, lose track of time) Drugs Aspirin Smoking	**Gross** Meat Cheese Eggs
Mobile (hyperactivity, exhaustion, insecurity, instability) Jumping Jogging Eating while doing other things	**Static** (sweet) Sweet porridge Sleeping during the day Quiet sitting
Clear (isolation, diversion) Too much cleansing (fasting, pancha karma, shanka prakshalana etc)	**Cloudy /sticky** Dairy Too much gluten

KAPHA GUNA (earth + water)	OPPOSITE GUNA
Heavy (weight gain, sleepiness, slow metabolism) Nuts/seeds beans sugar banana/dates wheat Meat, eggs, dairy	**Light** (bitter, pungent) Greens Raw food All vegetables Boiled or steamed
Slow (indigestion, dullness) Complicated food (too many ingredients) Rich food Fatty food	**Sharp** (pungent) Simple 3 ingredient food with spices Greens Raw radish
Cold (stagnation, unconsciousness, extra mucus, sore throat, low agni, low immunity)	**Hot** (pungent + sour) Chilli Lemon/ apple cider vinegar Arugula (rocket salad)
Oily (oily face, hair and faeces, slow metabolism) Fried Nuts Oil	**Dry** (bitter) Barley Buckwheat Corn Dry fruit and vegetables
Slimy (calm mind but in excess, passive mind) Dairy Too much gluten	**Rough** Broccoli Cauliflower Raw vegetables
Dense (overweight, heaviness, dense muscles) Meat Cheese Eggs	**Liquid** Juices Vegetable soups Bean soups Ginger tea

Soft (kindness but in excess, attachment)	Hard
Avocado	Raw apple
Banana	raw vegetables
Overcooked vegetables	Coral, metallic compounds
Static (attachment, oversleeping, inactivity)	Mobile
Sleeping after food	Waking up early
Lack of exercise	Not sleeping during the day
	Exercise
Sticky (attachment)	Clear
Wheat	Fasting
Rice	
Gross (obstruction, obesity)	Subtle
Meat	Sprouted seeds
Dairy	Raw greens
Eggs	Aromatic herbs

CHAPTER 8

Activated food
by Yogacharini Anandhi – Korina Kontaxaki
(Yoga Therapy with Yogacharya Jnandev 2022)

What is activated food?

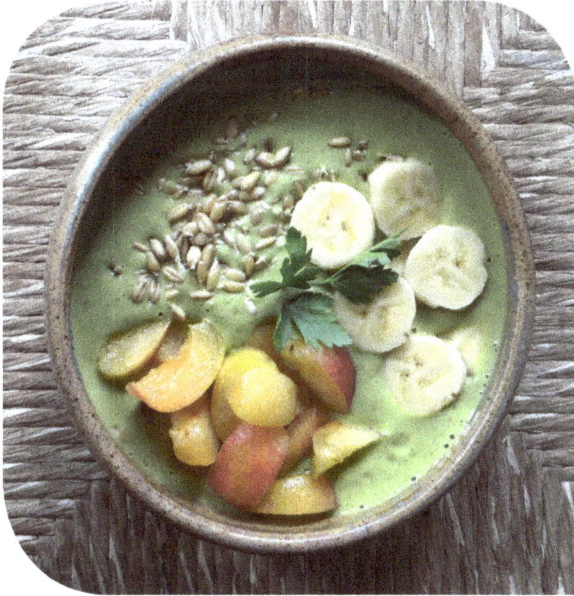

Activated food contains the prana needed for digestion and absorption
The Activated Diet has three main conditions:

1. Alive food (at least 95% fresh, raw or freshly cooked food).
   Maintaining high levels of vitality and retaining the nutrients of each food.
2. Easily digested (adding spice/herb formulas)
   Digestion will not tire the system and will encourage easier nutrient absorption (ama & agni)
3. In tune with the season and the environment (at least 80% local, seasonal ingredients).

Activated food gives us the most sustainable diet for the future. It also provides balance to the body, connecting it with the earth and the air.

The Yogic Diet is very close to the method of activated food, since both systems have the same goals:

❏ Ahimsa – no harm. Food that does not bring pain to any creature, man, animal or to the earth. In this way we do not burden our karma and we take care of the well-being and peace of ourselves and all around us.

❏ Diet that does not waste prana. It is very important when we practice meditation, but also when we have a very demanding life, that our food gives strength and energy to the body. To do this, food should not only be nutritious, but also sustain the energy/vitality in our system (body/emotions/mind). More than 90% of vitality is taken from the sun and breathing. Only 10% of vitality comes from food and this is because we use energy to digest our food. Only food that retains its natural energy from the sun, and is easy to digest, can sustain vitality for the body.

❏ Light, nutritious, healthy food. Yogic food must combine the above qualities so that one's health and strength enable them to evolve. And of course, the road to health and strength begins with our food.

❏ Sustainable living. Another piece of Ahimsa (no harm) that is omitted is the ability to be able to live with what exists, without requiring huge resources. Sustainable living is a must, especially these days where the population of the earth leaves no room for luxuries.

Alive food- What we add to our diet
- ❏ Sprouted seeds/legumes/grains
- ❏ Homemade plant-based milk
- ❏ Soaked seeds (rice, legumes, nuts, are eaten raw or cooked after we soak them in water for 6-8 hours)
- ❏ One raw meal a day (raw nuts, fruit, salads, dried fruits)

In the yogic diet we recommend 40% raw food and 60% freshly cooked food (in the summer we can reverse the percentages.)

Alive food - what we remove from diet:

- ❏ Canned food
- ❏ Pre-cooked food
- ❏ Artificial / processed (white pasta, bread from mass-producing bakeries, "fresh" packed juices etc.)
- ❏ Frozen food
- ❏ Microwave food
- ❏ Reheated food from yesterday
- ❏ Overcooked foods
- ❏ Food that is eaten a long time after cooking (4 hours or more)

Easily Digested - What habits we add to the diet

- ❏ Digestive formulas (try the classical digestive formula: cumin/chilli/turmeric/mustard seeds)
- ❏ Tridoshic tea (CCF Tea ; Koliandro / Cumin / Fennel)
- ❏ Mitahara: half full stomach
- ❏ Eat only when hungry
- ❏ Proper time distance between meals => new meal always on an empty stomach
- ❏ Right combinations. This essential element is very complicated and we must analyse and practice it in detail in another session.
- ❏ Hot water with lemon or apple vinegar every morning

Not Easily digested - What we take away from the diet

- ❏ Anything that makes us feel bad, bloated, heavy in the stomach - it's not for us!
- ❏ Excessive amount of carbohydrates. Replace carbohydrates with raw foods rather than with protein foods.

Food that is in tune
Does it grow in my local environment at the time of eating?

What we take away from our diet

- ❏ Fruit and vegetables out of season
- ❏ Fruits and vegetables from distant countries
- ❏ Seeds and fruits from distant countries that the body has experienced in our adult lives.

For more information you can take the complete Activated Vegan Food course, including practice and theory about the system:
How you get your protein with Activated Vegan Food
Digestive spice formulas
The real super food: sprouted legumes and seeds
Homemade, low-cost plant-based milk ready in just 5 minutes.
Bread, pasta, burgers and soups - the Activated way.
Replacement of dairy with super nutritious alternatives
Eating legumes without bloating
Tips for good digestion
Healthy cakes and desserts
Weekly meal preparation:
One-raw-meal-per-day,
One full vegan meal,
One light meal.

The above information is part of the Activated Vegan Food Seminar® by Anandhi Korina Kontaxaki.
You can find the full AVF guide here: https://yogalifewithanandhi.com/

CHAPTER 9

Fasting
by Yogacharini Anandhi

Why fast?

Fasting is one of the best techniques to reset the body/emotions/ mind and that's because the body makes its cells from the food we eat. The body is connected to the mind and emotions much more than we imagine. There are not only psychosomatics (when the mind affects the body) but also "somatopsychic" factors (when the body affects emotions). The lack of food makes the body "eat" itself. And what do you think has priority when this autophagy begins? Dead, diseased cells are eaten first. Thus, guided by the body, the mind/emotions/body system starts all over again, with its young, healthy cells.

Therefore, fasting

- 　　　　Sustains health
- 　　　　Is a Healing tool (because it resets the system)
- 　　　　Helps with Emotional/ Mind training
- 　　　　Is a spiritual training

It offers the following benefits:

- 　　　　Resting of the digestive organs
- 　　　　Freeing up energy to be used for healing and/or meditation
- 　　　　Improving agni (digestive fire)
- 　　　　Burning away ama (toxins)
- 　　　　Supporting a strong immune system.

*Read more about autophagy :
https://www.nobelprize.org/prizes/medicine/2016/press-release/

Who should fast?

Fasting is especially beneficial to:

Those suffering from obesity. Two main reasons that some people have bulimia are 1. A mainly mental habit is created: to eat often without the body to need it and 2. The cells that were fed and multiplied by excess food, ask for the same quality and quantity of food in order to survive.

Kapha conditions: One way to reduce mucus in the body is to "burn it" through the digestive fire, which increases through fasting.

Weak digestion: Fasting is the best way to strengthen the digestive fire. Another way to strengthen digestive fire is with special herbs/spices like fennel, ginger, pepper.

Intestine problems: (bacteria like e.coli, irritable colon, constipation). The best way to get rid of bad bacteria is to make them starve, removing their food. During fasting the harmful bacteria starve.

Too much ama (toxins): Fasting strengthens the digestive fire and this in turn "burns" the toxins.

Low on energy: The main reasons we have low energy are poor absorption by the intestine and toxins. Both are limited by fasting.

Uncontrolled emotions: The body is directly related to emotions and mind. When the body is uncontrollable, the same thing happens in the mind and emotions. When the body follows discipline, then the mind does the same.

> *"Fasting is the first principle of medicine;*
> *fast and see the strength of the spirit reveal itself."*
> Rumi

Ways to fast

1. Mono- fasting – eating one kind of food (ex. Kitchari*) one, two or three times per day.

2. Skipping a meal (Intermittent fasting) – keep the stomach empty for 12-16 hours

3. Raw food – eating only raw salads, vegetables, fruit, raw nuts, raw seeds and sprouted grains or sprouted pulses.

4. Fruit – raw fruit or one kind of fruit.

5. Juices

6. Water fasting – drinking only water for 24 hours

7. Dry fasting- not eating or drinking water for 24hours. This kind of fasting needs the supervision of an expert.

Fasting and Dosha
All Doshas can do mono-fasting with Kitchari and intermittent fasting

Vata
- Mono-fasting with Kitchari*
- Fasting with sweet fruit and warming teas (ginger, ginger+ fennel, coriander-cumin-fennel-black pepper tea)

Pitta
- Fruit fasting
- Raw food fasting
- Green juice fasting

Kapha
All kinds of fasting especially
- Sour fruit or juice fasting
- Honey and warm water fasting
- Black pepper and honey tea fasting

Duration
- 1 day regularly (once a week or twice a month) for sustaining health
- 1-3 days for healing mild health conditions

- 3-21 days for supporting the healing of a serious health contrition (only in a specially set up environment)

How to end the fast
- For mono fasting, intermittent fasting, raw food fasting and fruit fasting we can just eat something light for the first meal and then eat as normal.
- Break juice fasting with fruit
- Break water fasting with juice or fruit
- Break dry fasting with a banana or apple and then sip water slowly.

Who should ask their doctor or ayurvedic practitioner before fasting?
People with
- Low iron
- Low blood pressure
- Problems with blood sugar (diabetes) because they might feel extremely weak during fasting.

People with
- Heart problems
- Who are elderly
- With chronic illness because their body might not handle the lack of food.

Who should not fast
- Very young children (under 12 yrs)
- Very old people who didn't fast in the past
- Underweight or undernourished people
- Women who breastfeed

- Pregnant women
- People with ulcers

More about fasting
- Tea can be included in every method except dry fasting and water fasting
- If you have never fasted, start from No1.
- Chew food when fasting or when breaking the fast
- Avoid heavy foods after fasting (meat, fried food, roasted nuts, cheese and all saturated fat)
- Try not to eat more than usual after the fasting
- Eat slowly (slower than usual) so that you can check how much food you can digest

Conclusion
Consider :
- Health condition
- Prakrithi / Vikriti (dosha)
- Eating habits
before you suggest fasting for healing.
Generally speaking one day of mono-fasting or raw fasting for one day will assist any therapy.

*Kitchari = a combination of a grain and a legume and vegetables in a warm soup. The dish commonly uses whole grains and legumes like lentils.

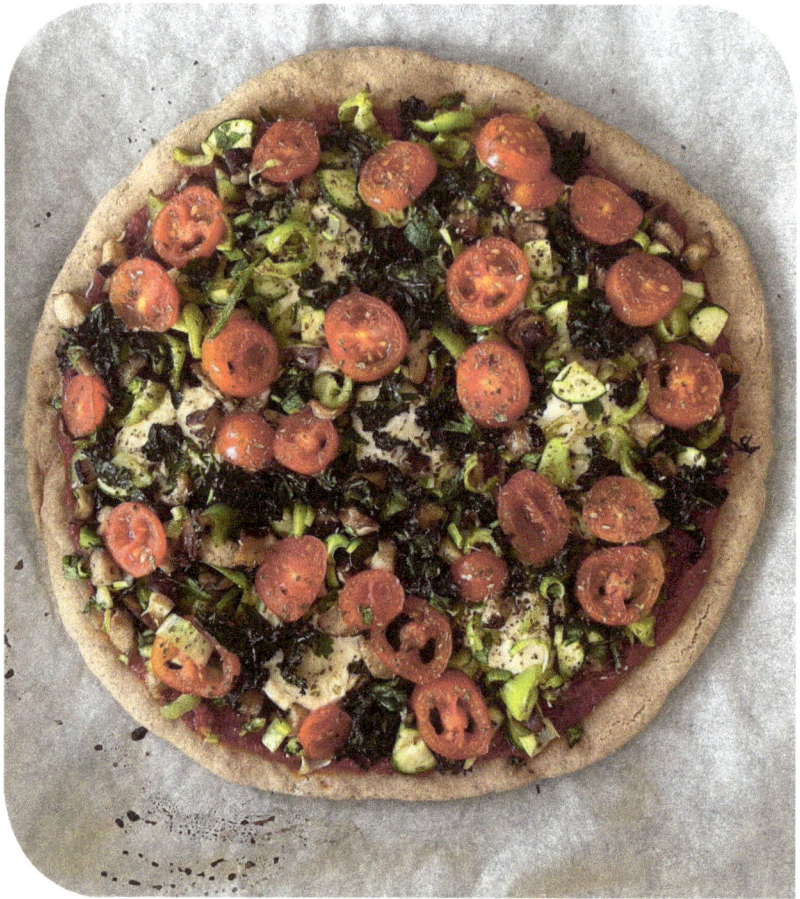

CHAPTER 10

A Yogi, Bhogi, Rogi and Drohi

by Yogachariya Jnandev Giri

Lord Krishna states that "A Yogi is the one who has the senses under control and is able to withdraw the mind from objects of senses or focus outward at his own will – just like a tortoise is able to extend or withdraw its limbs." Bhagavad Gita (2/58)

First self-enquiry is to find out if "you are a Yogi, Bhogi, Rogi or Drohi?

Yogi – One who has mastered the mind and remains in inner balance or tranquillity.

Bhogi – One who lives life for worldly consumerism.

Rogi – One who suffers some form of health issue.

Drohi – One who is against all the appropriate life habits.

These days the word Yogi or Yogini is quite often used as a title for anyone who practices yoga in some form, and they may even have no idea of what yoga really means other than a form of exercise.

The Himalayan yogis say that "Three people can occasionally sleep at night, they're: Yogi, Bhogi, and Rogi. "Yogi, because he is steadfastly engaged in Yoga Sadhana; Bhogi as they are addicted to material pleasures and ever engrossed in pleasing their senses and Rogi (once a Bhogi) who have abused their body and mind so much that it has resulted in pain and health issues resulting in suffering and misery, and they are therefore unable to sleep."

Only a true Yogi knows that the material objects can only bring temporary joy. Mastery of Ashtanga Yoga and one whose mind and senses are well established in the self in order to be united with the divine is the only source of absolute bliss – also known as Satchitadananda. This process of following the yogic path is known as Yoga Sadhana and the follower of Yoga is known as a Yoga Sadhaka or Sadhaki and not a Yogi or Yogini.

Ayurveda describes these four categories of people as follows, "One who eats once a day is a Yogi (mastered one). One who eats twice a day is a Bhogi (living for pleasure and consumerism). One who eats three times is a Rogi (one with ill-health). One who eats four times is a Drohi (destructive or troublemaker to society)."

This ancient concept of Ahara or Food consumption is not merely about the food itself. Yoga mentions that "worldly people out there with the attitude of a Bhogi (consumerism) are living to eat, consuming for pleasure while a Yogi is only eating and consuming what is necessary to live." This idea of Yogi, Bhogi, Rogi and Drohi in a true sense is about the attitude, mindset, habits and desires. We are not only hungry for food, but there is stronger hunger for other pleasure-seeking activities like sex, entertainment, social media, self-appraisal, attention, reward, ego, success, money, etc., leading us to all sorts of physical, mental, emotional, social and economic problems.

The quality of inner consumerism, media, information, associations, and so many other such activities we are taking part in can be easily looked at from the four types of personalities.

The innate appetite to gratify our senses and seek pleasure is very strong in all of us and can easily take over our Buddhi and Viveka. Our desire to feast our eyes on certain visions, our ears on certain sounds or music, our taste buds with certain flavours, our brain with certain intellectual ideas is unique and deep. We get cravings of certain touch and smell sensations. Our muscles can overindulge in a regime of extreme exercise and the mind can be captivated by certain ideas, thoughts, and words.

Many of us supress or over-consume unhealthy emotions such as resentment, revenge, jealousy, guilt and fear. Many people use harsh language, words and emotional torture to harm other people. Overconsumption of social media, an endless obsession with various conspiracy theories and negative attitudes are all part of Drohi or the destructive nature.

Our body and mind flourishes with a balanced approach to fulfilling our innate needs and desires whilst our health and wellbeing is destroyed when we overindulge, regardless of the object of our desires and due to our enchantment with such. Even excessive exercise, nutrition, or hatha yoga, etc. can become an addiction. Excess of any type of activity produces an inordinate amount of stress on the body and mind as well as taking away time which could be spent on withdrawing our senses inwards to digest the food, process the information, rest, sleep and enter into meditation.

Scientific research by Harvard Medical School shows the result of stress and overconsumption on our hippocampus, which is smaller in depressed people because stress can suppress the production of new nerve cells needed for its regeneration.

Even our obsession and excessive focus on physical health can lead to ill health and allow no time to enjoy or live our full potential. A healthy body (Swastha tan) is essential for our day-to-day life and spiritual quest. But still our attitude and mindset matters the most. As it is said, "pain may or may not exist in your life, it is not always in your control, but suffering is optional – we chose to suffer with a problem or deal with it and thrive towards better."

A Yogi refines and disciplines his cravings and passions, and follows the path of moderation (madhyam-marga or mitahara) in sensory gratification, no matter how delightful or tempting the experience in front of him. He eats just enough to live and does not let his cravings overwhelm him. He takes what is absolutely necessary to survive. He doesn't hold on to anything for the sake of the future and lives fearlessly in abundance.

We become Rogis when we chase a desire, hunger, thirst, goal, person, emotion, experience or desire without restraint and exert ourselves beyond our capacity and desire to attain them at any cost. This excessive single-mindedness usually is a result of some deep-seated psycho-emotional pain or blockage that we are unable to process and also maybe we are unaware of it. These emotions and desires urge us forward or hold us back and seem to have a life of their own. Our compulsions lead us to self-destructive behaviours that demolish our peace of mind and fuel further negative cravings.

Rogi in Sanskrit is also used to describe a person with some sort of health issue – a patient who is sick or diseased. These compulsive impulses raise our stress hormones and destroy or over-activate our sympathetic nervous system which destroys our peace of mind, affects our equanimity, homeostasis and the balance between our sympathetic and parasympathetic nervous systems.

In spiritual terms (adhyatmik) "a yogi who lives free from material attachment. A bhogi is the one who lives for material objects. A Rogi is one who solely identifies oneself with the body and the health of the body. We are Rogis when we identify solely with the body. A Drohi is the one who identifies the self as a victim and opposes the divine principles." A Bhogi is a passionate, goal-oriented person with strong opinions and often strong ambitions. They carry a great desire to succeed in life through material possessions, recognition, pride and/or wealth. Material satisfaction and validation through others is very important for these people.

According to Shawn Achor, the author of "Scientific Proof that Happiness is a Choice," every time we achieve success, our brain moves the goalpost of what success is.

A Drohi is someone who carelessly desires material possessions, power and egocentric recognition – all of which can be deadly and toxic. These will not only destroy his life but end up distressing others around him as well.

Yoga Vashistha, "A person who either eats too much or too less, who engages in stubborn bodily pleasures and is extreme in his emotional inclinations can rarely be a Yogi."

References and Resources:

1. https://www.health.harvard.edu/mind-and-mood/what-causes-depression
2. https://www.shawnachor.com
3. http://www.yogayuktalife.com/articles/2015/4/9/are-you-a-yogi-bhogi-or-rogi
4. https://www.vedic-management.com/yogi-bhogi-rogi/
5. Yoga Chiktisha By Dr Ananda Balayogi Bhavanani
6. Yoga Step By Step by Dr Swamiji Gitananda Giriji
7. Charaka Samhita -- PV Sharma Translator, Chaukhamba Orientalia, Varanasi, India, 1981, pp. ix-xxxii (I) 4 Volumes

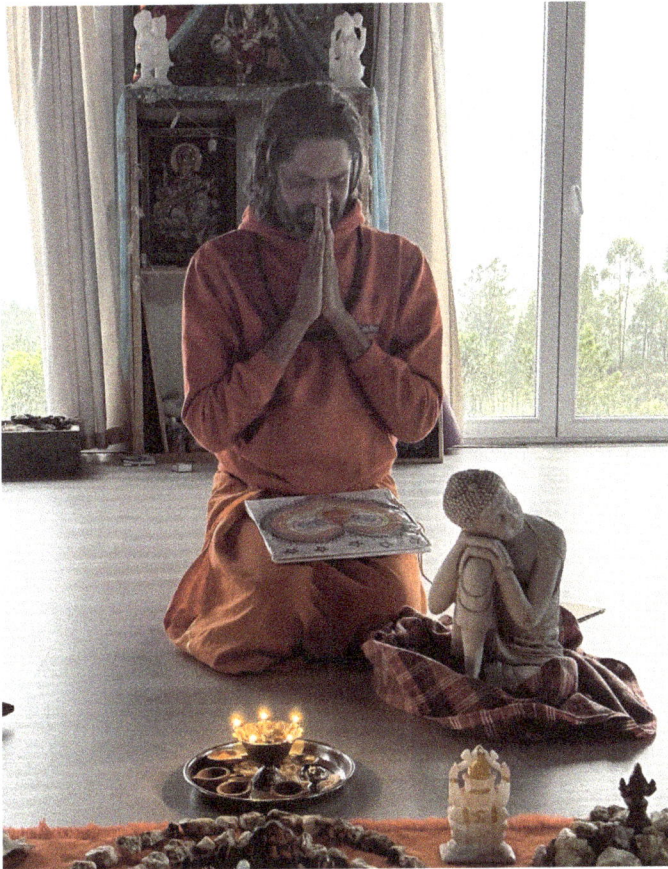

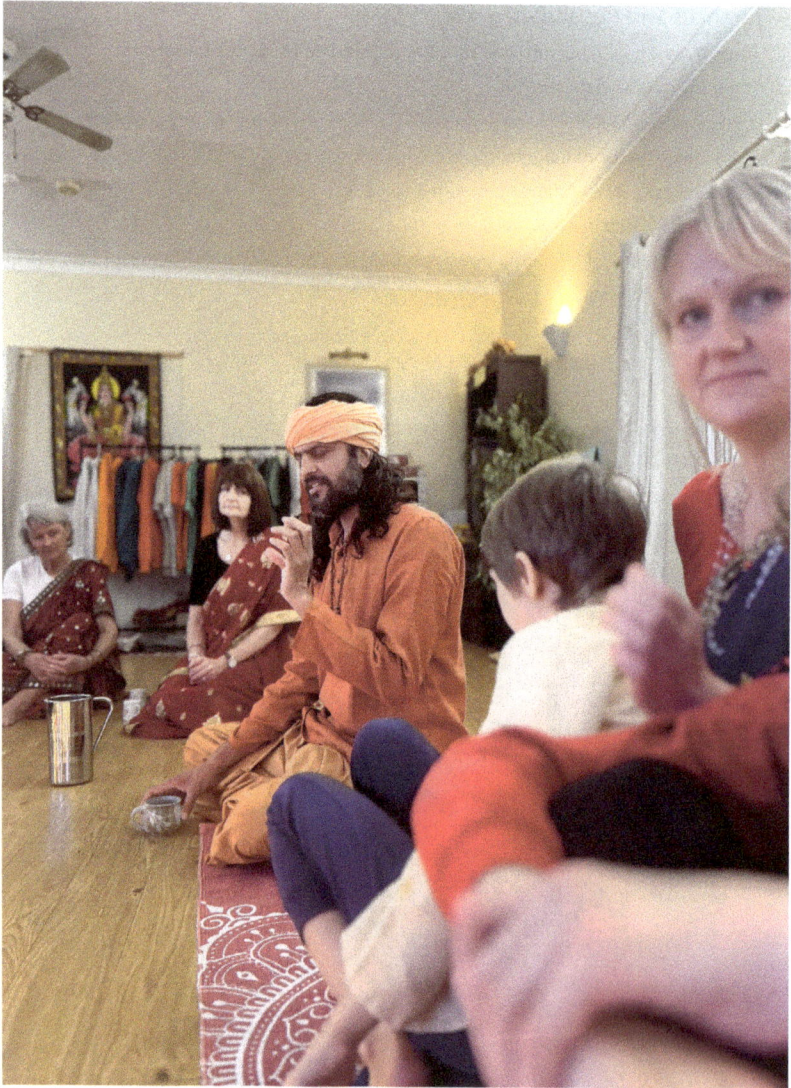

CHAPTER 11

Application of Dosha and Yoga Therapy Module

by Yogachariya Jnandev Giri

Step 1: Living Well in Harmony with Our Body, Mind and Constitutional Building Blocks

What, How & Why

This assessment is done by the individuals themselves as Yoga and Ayurveda describes how "the self is the most skilled, knowledgeable and wise authority on itself". Listening to your own body, or as a yoga therapist listening to care seekers' needs, has to be done in a unique way. Make sure you do your own assessment to understand your own body, your mind and vital energies.

This Dosha module should help you develop more self-awareness, self-knowledge and the understanding to be better equipped to deal with common signs and symptoms of imbalances and various health issues. The Yoga and dosha models together help us to understand how to heal our body, mind and energies with the easily available and accessible tools of hatha yoga, pranayama, mudras, relaxation practices, meditation, mantra, diet, and lifestyle modifications.

Yoga is a way of life and dosha a model of Ayurveda that together help us to develop the basic skills of diagnosis and understanding of health issues caused by imbalances and lifestyle factors.

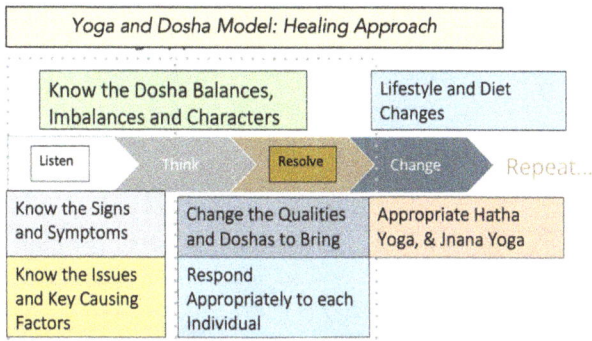

Yoga and Dosha Model: Healing Approach

Know the Dosha Balances, Imbalances and Characters		Lifestyle and Diet Changes
Listen	Think	Resolve	Change	Repeat...
Know the Signs and Symptoms	Change the Qualities and Doshas to Bring	Appropriate Hatha Yoga, & Jnana Yoga
Know the Issues and Key Causing Factors	Respond Appropriately to each Individual	

Your Basic Steps :
1. Try to know yourself or your care seeker.
2. Identify the issues and imbalances.
3. Identify the lifestyle, diet and other aggravating factors.
4. Introduce healthy changes like appropriate hatha yoga, pranayama, mudra, relaxation, diet changes, lifestyle changes.
5. Work gradually to change the qualities and constitution towards balance.
6. Motivate towards 3R's – REGULARITY, REPETITION & RHYTHM.

According to Lord Shiva "If the quality (guna) is there, the dosha is there."
-Shiva Samhita

Dhosha Imbalances and Health Issues

By using this table, you can identify Dosha imbalance in individuals you are working with. You can also support your outcomes by using the Dosha test if you wish to go deeper in your understanding and use of this model as part of yoga therapy.

PITA-RELATED IMBALANCES	FACTORS THAT AGGRAVATE PITA
• High Body Temperature • Health issues associated by excessive heat or redness • Indigestion, diarrhoea • Infectious diseases • Liver disorders • Ulcers, acidity • Skin rashes • Hypertension • Hyperthyroidism • Migraine headaches • Haemorrhoids • Vision disorders • Anger, irritability, jealousy • Becoming compulsive in routine • Seeking power and control • Rigid behaviour	• Chronic or intense stress • Pushing too hard at work • Insufficient and imbalanced exercise • Unrealistically high expectations of self or others • Excessive stimulants • Eating hot, spicy, or greasy foods • Heat and humidity

VATA-RELATED IMBALANCES	FACTORS THAT AGGRAVATE VATA
<ul><li>Pain, and inflammation in muscles and tissues</li><li>Impaired or abnormal movement</li><li>Deteriorating tissues</li><li>High and Low bursts of energy</li><li>Rheumatoid arthritis</li><li>Sciatica</li><li>backache</li><li>weak digestion</li><li>constipation</li><li>Menstrual related health issues</li><li>Insomnia</li><li>Depression</li><li>Feeling restless, unsteady and fearful</li><li>Cravings for starches and sweets</li><li>Feelings of inadequacy, low self-worth</li><li>Impulsiveness</li><li>Scattered thinking</li><li>Frenetic activity</li></ul>	<ul><li>Stress and strains of life</li><li>Unwanted Changes even if they are minor or positive minor</li><li>Travel, especially by air</li><li>Sensory over stimulation</li><li>Over exhaustion</li><li>Unhealthy diet habits like skipping meals</li><li>Eating too many raw, or cold foods</li><li>Improper sleep</li><li>Poor bedtime routine</li><li>Erratic work hours</li><li>Changing of the seasons</li><li>Cold, dry climate</li><li>Failure to express feelings of grief, loss, or fear</li></ul>

KAPHA-RELATED IMBALANCES	FACTORS: AGGRAVATING KAPHA
• Nasal and Respiratory Congestion • Sinus disorders • Excessive tissue growth • Health Issues Aggravated by dampness, cold and moisture • Weight gain, obesity • Oedema • Respiratory disorders like asthma • Diabetes • Impotence • Lethargy, fatigue • Benign tumours • Feeling sluggish and hopeless • Difficulty in mental focus • Memory problems • Excessive sleeping	• Chronic stress • Dull job • Meaningless or Lifeless relationship • Lack of movement • Excess sleep • Overeating • Too much sweet, salty, or fatty foods • Taking sedatives, like alcohol or sleeping pills • Relationships with excessive dependency and clinging • Too little or too much contact with others • Cold and damp weather • Lack of sunshine

We Must Understand

The energetic composition of our Doshas (VPK) have a positive or negative effect on our body, mind, senses, energy, perception and personality.

- What may be bad for vata, may be good for kapha and vice versa. In this way what a vata person may feel is appropriate may be totally unacceptable to a pitta or kapha person.
- What may be intense for one person may not be intense for another. Like Vata may make us more sensitive, whilst kapha may

make us more accepting.
- Our perceptions are dependent upon our nature, qualities and constitutions (prakriti, guna & dosha).
- Each Dosha has its beneficial quality as well as health issues associated with the imbalances.

Our Feelings, Thoughts, Mind and Doshas

Yoga and Ayurveda principles are based on natural healing principles and practices for healing our body, mind and soul. So this is more of a lifestyle or a way of life then just another therapeutic tool. Anyone can learn these sets of principles and practices and follow them in day-to-day life to regain health and wellness along with connecting with our true nature. One of the most beautiful and profound practice in Yogic Awareness is to be aware or feel your true feelings. We just need to feel our innate and true feelings and work on reorganising our body, mind and intelligence to become our better self. Our feelings, emotions and thoughts directly influence our neurobiology, qualities (gunas) and constitution (dosha).

Checking our Current State:-
Where am I now in the context of my energetic state?
What kinds of feelings and thoughts am I going through now?
What is going through my mind now?
What signs and symptoms of imbalances do I feel now?

Now try to answer the following questions:

(1) What emotions have I been feeling lately?

(2) How would I describe my state of mind lately?

Doshas & The Symptoms of Excess Chart

Quick Self Assessment - mind & emotions

Signs of Vata Excess	Signs of Pitta Excess	Signs of Kapha Excess
trouble sleeping indecision overwhelm anxiety restlessness difficulty focusing difficulty completing tasks Interrupted thoughts cycling emotions Impulsivity addictive tendencies tired- empty tank	irritability intensity overanalysis (self) criticism impatience quick temper aggression confrontation focus on problems overworking get it done mode	sluggish mind sleepiness tired - heavy Stubbornness Resistance to change Emotional baggage melancholy easy to cry Lack of motivation tough am wake

Quick Self Assessment - body

Signs of Vata Excess	Signs of Pitta Excess	Signs of Kapha Excess
Gas bloating or belching Constipation or straining Small, or hard stools Get full quickly dryness- skin, hair, nails pain stiffness inability to sit still Cold hands and feet frequent urination	heartburn frequent or loose stools Inflamed colon feeling hot Acne skin redness or irritation Inflamed, tense muscles Infection anywhere	heaviness Slow sluggish digestion low am appetite fluid retention bloating Weight gain congestion Excess Sweat Oily skin or hair Swollen ankles

Vata Energy	Pitta Energy	Kapha Energy
Degenerating Stimulating Moving Changing Entropic *Too Much* ↓ Depletion Degeneration Irregularity	Working Digesting Transforming Producing Catabolic *Too Much* ↓ Inflammation Infection	Building Growing Nourishing Grounding Anabolic *Too Much* ↓ Accumulation Stagnation Blockage

Using some of these tables and information by Yogacharini Anandhi try to identify common signs & symptoms of imbalance then answer the following questions:

What signs of Vata excess are you currently experiencing? _____

_____

What signs of Pitta excess are you currently experiencing? _____

_____

What signs of Kapha excess are you currently experiencing ? _____

_____

You can follow this separately for body, mind, emotions and energy.

Category	Vata Signs deficiency, irregularity, degeneration	Pitta Signs inflammation, infection, heat	Kapha Signs accumulation, stagnation, congestion, growth	
Emotional Body	overwhelm anxiety & worry hypersensitive extreme emotion internal conflict cycling emotions	irritable impatient short-tempered angry jealous resentful	sad want to be alone psych. baggage holding on to grudges depression crying	
Mind	reactive trouble sleeping indecision restlessness difficulty focusing difficulty completing racing thoughts impulsive choices addictive tendencies	intense focus on problems activated to solve overworking pressured to-do list mania overanalyzing (self) critical impatient righteous	unmotivated unclear dull stubborn unmotivated tough a.m. wakeup	

NONPHYSICAL SUBTOTAL	_____	_____	_____
Digestion	gas, gurgling, bloating belching cramping, spasm constipation dry, small stools straining low appetite	hyperacidity increased appetite > 2 BMs/day loose stools narrow stools mouth sores	sluggish digestion poor a.m. appetite low physical hunger mucus in stool nauseous in a.m. heavy after eating	
Immunity & Blood	low immunity allergies food sensitivities cold hands and feet feeling cold	feeling hot flushed face, ears headaches- tension gout herpes outbreaks	not temperature-sensitive elevated blood sugar swollen feet/ hands	
	headaches - vasospasm	Inflammation tendency		
Skin	dry, flaky discolored, dull blackheads dry, itchy skin dry cuticles	red undertone inflamed red acne rash or hive prone	smooth oily whiteheads deep acne cysts	
Sinuses & Respiration	dry, cracked lips dry sinus membranes runny nose dry throat dry, itchy eyes	sinus infection bloody nose/ mucus respiratory allergies	congestion a.m. phlegm post nasal drip clogged ears headaches - sinus pressure	
Nerves & Adrenals	trouble sleeping dark circles under eyes	spend a lot of time in "get-it-done" mode	slow responses over sleepy weight gain	
Muscles, Joints & Mobility	pain stiff creaky joints worse in a.m. tremor unsteadiness in movement	inflamed muscles and joints worse after use	swollen ankles swollen, cool joints joint pain with rain slow movement	
Kidneys & Urination	urinary frequency	frequent urinary tract infections	Bladder/kidney stones Cloudy urine	
Sexuality & Reproduction	extreme sexual frequencies and practices after time, no libido dry tissues irregular menses uterine cramping	frequent yeast infections with burning STDs	slow to rise libido, sluggish orgasm excessive discharge yeast infections with less symptoms heavy menses dark, clotted menses fibroids, polyps ovarian cysts enlarged prostate	
PHYSICAL SUBTOTAL	_____	_____	_____	

CHAPTER 12
Dhatus, Mallas and Dosha
by Yogachariya Jnandev Giri

If and when the three doshas are balanced, they support each other's functions and the body maintains a state of health and wellness. The appropriate proportion of each dosha as per the proportion by the innate nature is known as dosha-samya. If it increases or decreases, it is known as doshavaishamya. So while studying the body, one's health or ill health, it is important to understand and analyse doshas. After the three doshas, one has to consider dhatu and malla.

It is stated that "Doshadhatumalamulam hi shariram", which means "dosha, dhatus or tissues and mallas or waste products make up our body and health."

Vakbhata has the following reference:
Vayuh pittam kaphascheti trayo doshah samasatah | V S 1.6
Vikruta vikruta deham ghananti the vardhayanticha | V S 1.7
The body contains three doshas – kapha, pitta, vata. When they are imbalanced, they destroy life. When they are balanced, they manifest good life and health.

Ras, Rakta, Mans, Med, Asthi, Majja and Shukra are seven dhatus. These are also known as substances.
Urine, stools and sweat are known as malla. They are also substances and can be affected by the doshas.
Ras (Fluids) - This is a liquid or fluid, flowing dhatu. The Panchmahabhootas and ayurvedic diet should include six rasas, twenty characteristics and all types of viryas in balance. Further when the food is digested properly with the help of digestive fire in the stomach, the nutritious substance generated, which has a subtle essence, is known as rasa. Its place is the heart and that is circulated through all the vessels of the body with the support of the Vyana Vayu. Other dhatus are then made from the rasa.

Rakta (Blood) - When the rasa rich with Jala or water reaches the liver and the spleen, it is converted into Rakta or Blood which is red in colour due to the Ranjak Pitta. The blood in Panchamahabhautic people exhibits the characteristics of Prithvi, Aap, Tej, Vayu and Aakash in that order and has a peculiar smell, liquidity, red colour, flow and voidness. When the blood is washed away from a cloth and does not leave any stain on the cloth, it is termed as healthy blood (defectless).

Mansa (Muscular Tissue or flesh) - With the supporting blood, the fire (agni) in the muscular tissue operates in the mansvah strotra and mansa dhatu is produced. The warmth or heat of the Vayu and Tej is mixed up in the blood and it becomes thick. It gets ripened due to the fire of the mansa and takes the form of mansa. The cells and the muscles in the body are also various forms of flesh. These muscles protect the organs and support their functions. The muscles bear the weight of the body. The joints move. All these movements are operated by the Vyana Vayu.
Med (Adipose Tissue)- With the support of mansa (flesh), the fire in the med operates in medovah strota and the dhatu med is created. It provides strength to the body.

Asthi (Bones) - From the Panchmahabhutas in the supporting elements, the fire (agni or tej) in the asthidhatu operates and creates toughness. This creates bones. Due to Vayu, they can be porous. This function is carried on in asthivah strota.

Majja (Bone Marrow) - Asthidhatu supporting majja gets operated upon by the fire in majja in majjavah strota, and majja dhatu is created. This resides in the cavities in the bones and is known as majja.

Shukra (Generative Tissue) - Shukra dhatu is produced from majja with the union of tej or fire. The origin of shukra dhatu is in shukradhar kala in shukravah strota all over the body. Though the testicles and the ovaries are the main origins, shukra dhatu is produced all over the body in a miniscule form. It drizzles in the testicles.

The shukra dhatu originating in the female body is known as Aartava, which are of two kinds:

1. Bahihpushpa – This aartaya is produced in the uterus (Garbhasaya) each month. This is not useful for conceiving (Garbha-Dharna), but very much necessary for purification of the uterus (Garbha-Suddhi).

2. Antarpushpa – This second form of aartaya is produced in the uterus in a very tiny form each month. This takes part in conception by absorption of Shukra (semen).

Ojas – This is the brilliance or subtle excellent glow or energy in the Shukra Dhatu of all the seven Dhatus. The heart is the seat of Ojas, and it pervades the whole body. It is the fundamental energy principle in all living beings and our state of health and well-being depends on it. Prana dwells through this energy. This can be considered the eighth Dhatu or spiritual subtle energy field.

There are upadhatus for all sapta dhatus, which are:
- Rasa - Stanya and Raj
- Rakta - Kadara and Shira
- Mansa - Vasaa and Twacha
- Meda - Snayu, Sandhibandha, Shira
- Mala – waste products of which there are three.

Purish (faeces) - Once the food has been fully digested, at the time of division of Sarkitta, Purish is produced by Purishdharakarla in Purishvah Strota. According to Charaka, the measure of it is 7 handfuls. Vayu and Agni are outcomes and governing principles (dharana).

Mutra (Urine) - According to Charaka, the measure is 4 handfuls.
Sweda (Perspiration) - This is mal of meda and released through the skin. It plays an important role in keeping the skin and hair moist and maintaining body temperature.

(Ayurveda Explains Conception and Fetal Body Development)
Once we understand the principles of tridosha, saptadhatu and Malas, we should try to understand the concept of the physical body according to Ayurveda.

Vayu provokes the teja in the body due to the friction caused between male and female genitals during coitus. Due to the union of male and female Tejas and Vayu, the male shukra begins flowing and gets dislocated from the testicles and enters the vagina through the penis. The semen or shukra gets united with the aartaya or egg there.

Union of Raj in the form of fire or Tejas, and shukra in the form of soma, form the fetus, moving into the uterus and growing there until the time of birth.

Vayu separates from the fetus in the forms of Chaitanya, doshas, dhatus, Mala and other organs. Teja or fire governs the digestion. Gradually the foetus develops hands, legs, a tongue, ears, nose and other organs to take form in the body.

Ayurveda describes the fetal body development in the womb in four states as follows-

- ❏ In the first stage the shape of the body is developed with Asthi (bones) and Mansa (muscles) dhatus.
- ❏ In the second phase Prakriti or nature of the body is developed, which includes inner organs and internal processes. Rasa, Rakta, Meda, Majja and Shukra development takes place in this phase.
- ❏ Vikriti or disturbance in doshas, dhatus, and malas may develop in phase three.
- ❏ Nishkruti means the process of examining the body with the respective Vikriti which happens in the fourth phase. (Note: third and fourth phases are to be studied as part of Ayurveda Specialist Practitioner Courses)

CHAPTER 13

Asthi Dhatu: Ayurveda and Yogic Perspectives

by Yogachariya Jnandev Giri

Asthi means bone or structural support. The asthi dhatu gives solid structure to the body. As part of Annamaya Kosha or the physical body, asthi dhatu is formed as posaka (unstable) medas dhatu, which flows into the purisha dhara kala and is digested by the Asthi-Agni. In addition to the formation of the bones, teeth and the upasthu or secondary tissue are formed through this process. The hair and nails are described as the waste products (malas) of this metabolic process.

The purisha dhara kala is the membrane that holds the asthi agni. Purisha means "faeces". The term is also used to describe the large intestine as in the purishavaha srota. This establishes a connection between large intestines, bones and health. The large intestine is the primary seat of the vata dosha. The close relationship between these two tissues enables us to understand the connection of the health issues of the bones and muscles in relation to vata dosha imbalance. When there is a health issue in the large intestine (gas, constipation, lack of healthy gut bacteria), this can lead to bone and muscle problems like osteoporosis, arthritis, and bones may become more porous and air filled.

Bones are primarily made up from a solid structure known as Prathvi Bhuta or earth element. Space between the solid matter is filled by Vayu or the wind element. This helps bones to be solid and structurally strong but also light so as to support easy movement. Long and hollow bones are filled with hematopoietic tissue known as bone marrow or Majja Dhatu.

The low asthi agni leads to excess production of asthi dhatu. This results in production of denser tissue. Those with excess of Kapha, having low agni, will have production of thicker and denser bones.

People with pitta nature will have high agni, which results in less dense asthi majja which are metabolically more active. This may lead to narrow and weak bones, as well as inflammation of pitta is lessened.

Vata nature leads to a variable agni which causes the lesser production of asthi dhatu. This results in poorer quality of bones, which can be thinner and more fragile.

Ayurveda recommends that to produce healthy asthi dhatu, one must consume adequate amounts of prithvi and vayu bhutas through a balanced diet. Prathvi is present in abundance in sweet foods (madhuriya ahara) such as grains and nuts as well as astringent foods like beans and lentils.

Vayu is present in bitter and pungent foods like most vegetables. Most of us should be consuming these foods as part of a healthy diet already but Ayurveda mentions that consumption alone does not guarantee production of healthy asthi. These two elements must be properly digested so that their qualities can lead to production of healthy bones.

The jatharagni (the primary digestive fire) must be healthy and balanced. If the jatharagni is out of harmony even healthy food will lead towards production of ama, which causes toxicity of the body and mind.

Asthi Dhatu and Health Issues

Over active Vata leads to weak and fragile bones, that can become osteoporotic and fracture easily.

Pitta over-activation leads to bone infections (osteomyelitis) and inflammation.

Over-active Kapha leads to excessively thick and dense bones.

Osteoarthritis is a combination of vata-kapha imbalance condition in which vata (motion, stress and ageing) causes irregular growth in an unhealthy manner, leading to bone spurs.

Rheumatoid arthritis is a Sannipatika condition, where Vata irritates

Kapha to cause irregular bone growth. Vata blows the wind to the Pitta causing inflammation and bone deterioration. Ama or toxins work as a supporting aid to this situation.

The Asthi Dhatu and Manas or Psychology

Ashti Dhatu plays an important role in the structural composition of our body, but it also plays an important role in our mental and emotional composition. The way we stand, walk, sit, and hold our posture is a physical expression of our mental and emotional state. One's posture or Asana is not just the gesture of physical posture, but also the quality and state of their mind and inner self.

Maharishi Patanjali refers to Asana or Gesture as "sthirum sukham asana", which means "state of being at ease and stable with and within ourselves and composure." This statement clearly refers to the connection between our structural posture, gesture and the state of our inner self.

If our asthi dhatu is weak and fragile, there will always be a struggle in standing firm and composed in the face of adversity or controversy. There will be a lack of steadfastness.

When the asthi dhatu is healthy and strong, there is a sense of healthy confidence, stability, confidence and ability to make clear decisions and follow one's own beliefs and ideas.

If there is an excess of asthi dhatu, the quality of the prathvi element is increased, which leads that individual to become overly attached, obstructive and stubborn. For these people it is very difficult to move forward or change direction in life.

When there is a deficiency of asthi dhatu, the quality of Prathvi element is decreased and there will be very little attachment or stability in life's activities and choices. These people can be easily persuaded by others and lack their own will.

Kapha dosha causes an excess in asthi dhatu, Vata dosha leads towards to deficiency in asthi dhatu. In the long term Pitta dosha burns down asthi dhatu resulting in a weak and fragile body and mind.

Asthi Dhatu and Chakras

In the Pranamaya Kosha, health of asthi dhatu relies on healthy prana flow through the Mooladhara Chakra. Prana flowing through this chakra is associated with the qualities of the Prathvi element in the pranamaya kosha and manifests in solidity, stability, strength and endurance of body and mind. This develops a solid sense of Self (Atma-Nistha).

The Manipura Chakra is associated with the Agni element, Anahata Chakra is associated with the Vayu element, while Vishuddha Chakra is associated with qualities of the Akash element. Through these Chakras, the qualities of the respective elements and prana vayus are circulating or governed. If there is an excess flow of pranic energy currents through these chakras, it will also increase the qualities of respective elements, which in excess will cause weakening of asthi dhatu in both the physical and mental bodies.

Asthi Dhatu and Health Assessment

Assessment of asthi dhatu directly is not possible as it covered by mansa dhatu (flesh and muscles) and tvacha (skin). But we can assess the asthi dhatu by means of upadhatus and malas. By examining the hair, nails, and teeth, a Yoga Practitioner can determine the state and health of asthi dhatu.

If there is a deficiency and weakness of asthi dhatu, hair density becomes scant and weak. Hair loss and scalp irritation may be distributed throughout or in patches. Also, nails will become weak and break easily. The teeth will also become crooked, darker or grey compared to usual. These findings are also associated with Vata dosha.

An excess of asthi dhatu, hair density becomes full and crowded. The nails will be thick, and the teeth become large, straight and whiter. These are signs of Kapha dosha in the asthi dhatu. Kapha disorder also leads to sluggish digestion and a stubborn mind. When these are seen together in the care seeker, then Kapha dosha has entered into asthi dhatu too.

When the Pitta dosha has affected the asthi dhatu, the teeth and nails will become pale in shades of yellow and the hair will lose its colour and turn grey. Gradually this will lead to weaker nails and the hair will fall out.

Prevention, and Healing of Asthi Dhatu

Preservation of Asthi Dhatu and its wellness is easier to healing. Panchamahabhuta therapy (Naturopathy in Indian Ancient Therapies), Hatha Yoga, Healthy Diet, and Balanced Polarity and Chakras can be key practices in prevention and healing of asthi dhatu.

In order to heal the asthi dhatu, you will need to restore the balance of the Pancha-Mahabhutas especially between Prathvi and Vayu as well as balanced flow of the prana vayus Mooladhara, Manipura, Anahata and Vishuddha Chakra. The appropriate quantity ratio of these subtle elements varies with each individual's constitution.

Individuals with Kapha constitution will naturally have strong asthi dhatu. In these people deficiency of asthi dhatu is less likely than excess. Those with the Vata constitution will naturally tend to have a lower amount of asthi dhatu and are more susceptible to deficiency of asthi dhatu.

Individuals with Pitta constitution tend to have a moderate quantity of asthi dhatu and are only prone to deficiency when exposed to excess agni or heat for an extended period. In these individuals, asthi dhatu is affected adversely by vata imbalance too.

Asthi Dhatu and Diet

When the Vata Dosha is affecting the asthi dhatu, one needs to increase the quantity of Prathvi element in their diet. Prathvi is found in large amounts in sweet foods like grains, nuts, lentils and beans and lesser amounts in root vegetables. Fruits and leafy vegetables carry the least amount of Prathvi element. In naturopathy, mud baths, steam baths and hot and cold showers are highly recommended.

For people with Kapha Dosha affecting the asthi dhatu, it is important to decrease the quantity of Prathvi element in their diet and increase the Vayu element. Fruits and leafy vegetables and salads carry excess amount of the Vayu element. It is also important to note that too many fruits may aggravate the Jala aspect of Kapha and hence caution should be taken in terms of the quantity of fruits and vegetables consumed. The pungent and bitter foods are highly recommended to increase the quality of Vayu element. Increase in use of spices and a comparatively light diet is advisable.

If Pitta is affecting the asthi dhatu, it is advisable to decrease the quality of Agni element. The recommended diet should be one that is cooling and contains a reduced quantity of hot spices and cooked oils. Whole milk, wheat and other grains are recommended in moderate amounts. Beans and lentils are also recommended if they are easily digestible and not causing wind related issues in individuals.

Hatha Yoga, Yoga Vyayama and the Asthi Dhatu

Any form of healthy exercise increases the asthi-agni, which supports formation of high quality bones and supporting tissues. We need to be very careful with people with weak asthi dhatu as their bones and supportive muscles are weak and easily prone to fracture and damages due to a lack of endurance and strength. For people with weak bones, and structural issues like various types of arthritis, a gentle and slower form of hatha yoga or yoga vyayama should be considered as a healing practice and avoid vigorous and weight bearing exercises.

Walking in nature is one of the most healthy exercises as well as Panchamahabhuta therapy as you will be exposed to all the healthy elements of nature. Also water-based exercises can be a great way to start in people with more severe health issues related to bones and supportive tissues.

Short sessions of gentle hatha yoga vyayam suitable to each individual several times a day can be highly beneficial – especially isometric or static stretches (held between 10 seconds to 3 minutes) which can be a great way to stimulate the muscles, increase blood circulation and activate nerves to stimulate the healing process and reduce pain. Some of these yoga-based exercises can be very simple, here are few examples:
- Press your hands against each other in Namaskar Mudra and hold for few deep breaths.
- Clasp your fingers and pull them against each other to create tension and hold for few deep breaths.

- Stretch your feet away from the body and raise your arms over your head and stretch the arms upward and hold for few deep breaths.
- Press your shoulder against the wall and breathe deeply.
- Press both your arms against the wall and hold it for several deep breaths.
- Come to half plank or full plank and hold for a few breaths.
- Perform Janusirasana and hold the gentle stretch for a few breaths.
- Join the soles of your feet together in Baddha Konasana with knees pressing down, bring your hands in Garuda Mudra and hold the stretch for few deep breaths.

Other gentle hatha yoga kriyas can be introduced for further healing, enhanced blood circulation, cleansing, healthy pranic energy flow, and activating healing response like:
- Plavini Kriyas for legs, arms and neck along with neuroplasticity and healthy pranic flow.
- Brahma Mudra Kriyas for neck and shoulders
- Setu Bandha and Kati Chakra Kriyas for spine, hips, abdominal and pelvic areas.
- Rishikesh Suriya Namaskar for healthy body, mind and pranic energy.

A healthy pressure on joints, bones and muscles in an appropriately designed yoga session for care seekers can be a great aid to enhance health and wellness.

An appropriate pranayama and yogic relaxation should always follow hatha yoga or yoga vyayama for the optimum benefits.

Mantra Chanting, and Meditation for Healthy Asthi Dhatu

Meditation, mantra chanting, and spiritual contemplations enhance the coherence between pancha-koshas, pancha-bhutas, pancha-prana-vayus and chakras and hence develop a healthy body, mind and psyche. If possible sadhakas should follow meditation and mantra chanting on the floor as opposed to being on a chair as it brings us closer to earth and enhances the qualities of the Prathvi element. Focusing on Mooladhara chakra and its connection with the earth element also helps enhance the health and wellness of asthi dhatu.

One can follow Sukha Purvaka Pranayama (inhale for 6 x hold in for 6 x exhale for 6 x hold out for 6 counts; it can be followed in counts of 4, 6 or 8) for enhancing the qualities of the earth element and root chakra. One can also meditate on the earth mandala, which is a square or cube form of visualisation at the Mooladhara Chakra. This mandala is vibrant yellow in colour and can help with developing a greater sense of clarity, grounding, and stability. This supports the asthi dhatu.

One can chant the Bija Mantra LANG for the Mooladhara Chakra, or Pranava OM for complete physical, mental and psychic wellbeing, or OM SHANTI SHANTI SHANTI OM for inner peace and tranquillity.

Mantras can be chanted out loud, softly or mentally.
If the asthi dhatu is in excess, then dharna (concentration) and dhyana (meditation) can help enhance the qualities of Akasha (voidness or ether) and Vayu (wind) and hence will help purify excess of asthi dhatu. Further meditation on Anahata Chakra and Vishuddha Chakra can help cleanse and reduce the excess of asthi dhatu. Chanting of Bija Mantras for Anahata (YUNG) and Vishuddha (HUNG) can be a great aid to enhance the qualities of Akasha and Vayu and reduce excess of asthi dhatu.

Ayurveda and the Skeleton System

Ayurveda describes the skeleton system as the main basis of the human body, which includes skeleton and bones. It states that all the parts, organs and functions are supported by the Asthi (bone). Bones primarily belong to the Prathiv or solid element and are described as hard and durable. Even when the body is burnt on the pyre, all the bones do not get burned easily.

In traditional and Sanatan anatomy study Ancient Rishi and Ayurveda pioneer Sushruta describes the human body in six aspects. The torso and head are considered as the main part (mukhya sarira bhaga) while the two hands and two legs are considered to be the four branches. It is further described that as hands and legs are only branches, it is just like the branches of a tree. Even if the branches are cut, a tree stays alive as long as the main trunk and roots are there, so does our body stays alive even if the hands and legs are cut.

The upper and lower part of the body have 30 bones each. In the middle part of the body, the spinal cord is considered as primary. It is composed of 33 vertebrae, which are joined with each other. The seven vertebrae in the upper part of the spine are considered as part of the neck, followed by 12 as part of the chest. These are also known as ribs and termed as Parshuram or Varki in Sanskrit. The spinal cord is described like bamboo, thick at the base and narrowing as it grows upwards. It is also described as hollow inside through which the spinal cord or Nadis pass.
In the skull or head (kapal), there is a cavity made of eight flat bones. The brain is placed safely in this cavity, very well protected. The bones below the bones in the skull are known as Shankasthi. They are thin and beneath them there is a large number of blood vessels supplying blood to the brain.

In front of this cavity, there are 14 bones in the face. The cavity of the ears has a chain of small bones and hearing is carried through this chain of bones and nerve fibres.

According to Sushruta, there are 300 bones altogether and according to Charaka there are 360 bones. In a way it can be understood by understanding the way the bones are being counted or considered as part of our modern anatomy. Physiology describes 206 bones all together in a grown up adult.

These bones are grouped in six categories:-
Nalikasthi - These are long like tubes and hollow from within. They are stuffed with majja. Till the age of 20 years, the colour of this is red, then it turns yellow. These types of bones are in the hands and legs.

Kapalasthi - These are flat in nature. The above and below layer is separated and hollowed parts are made. Red majja fills it.

Valayasthi - These are round in shape. The ribs of the chest are of this type.

Tarunashthi - These are soft in nature. They are mainly in between the joints of the vertebrae; in between two vertebrae there is a circle of tarunasthi. Hence, any jolt to the body, till it reaches the brain, becomes mild.

Ruchakasthi - The teeth which are different from all the other bones in the body are covered under this. They are 28 or 32 in all.

Aanvashti - The bones which are smaller and irregular in size and which do not fit under any of the above categories fall under this. These bones have fat with blood.

Further, the entire bone system is divided into two main parts:-
Bahyakankal- the nails and teeth are considered in external bones as they don't have an outer layer of flesh and skin (mansa and tvach). These bones can be referred to as part of a diagnosis including the colour and structure of the nails and teeth.

Antahkankal- These are internal bones covered by flesh and bones.

All the bones are joined with each other, and these joints are known as Sandhi. Sandhis are classified as two categories:-
Sthir or Achal Sandhi - these are fixed joints like joints in the skull, jaw and teeth etc.

Chala or Cheshthavanta - These are movable joints. These joints and associated bones are covered with tarunasthi, which are elastic in nature and can withstand pulling and pushing. Sandhikosha is another layer above the tarunasthi which covers the joints like a bag. Inside these bags rests the grease-like substances known as shleshak and shleshma to support smooth movement.

Ayurveda describes eight types of sandhis :
Kor - Joints in the fingers, the wrists, the ankles and elbows.
Ulukhal - The joint of the thigh, joint at the roots of teeth.
Samugad - Joints near the shoulder, anus, reproductive organs, hips etc.
Pratar - Joints like neck, vertebrae of the back etc.
Tunnasevani - Joints of the kapalashthi at the face, waist etc.
Vaayastund - Joints near the chin on both sides.
Mandal (round) - joints at heart, eyes etc.
Sankhavarta – Joints in shape of circles at the ears, shankha (inner ear) etc.
Ayurveda describes 210 joints altogether.

Muscles and Ayurveda in Summary
Muscles join all the bones with each other and the movement is made with expansion and contraction of the muscles.
The muscles are of four types:
Pratanvarti Muscles - Four branches and in all joints
Vruta - Kandara - All round muscles
Sushira - Contracting muscles in big intestine
Pruthul (flat muscles) - muscles at side, chest, back, head etc

CHAPTER 14

Yoga, Ayurveda and Digestive Health
by Yogachariya Jnandev Giri

In Ayurvedic principles of health and understanding of diseases, as well as therapeutic processes, our digestive system plays a very important role. Ayurveda explains that the food we eat, the digestive process, the distribution and metabolic processes are all considered very important. Also in Yogic principles our mind, emotions and sense of wellbeing is connected with our solar plexus and sacral chakra. I am sure we all are familiar with the feeling of an upset or churning stomach during stressful, anxious or fearful times. Yoga and Ayurveda give an immense amount of importance to our digestive health. It is said that "being able to enjoy the meals you like itself is a blessing."

According to Ayurveda, there are seven constitutional tissues or aspects in the body:
- Rasa Dhatu: Plasma and fluid
- Rakta Dhatu: Blood
- Mamsa Dhatu: Muscles
- Medhas Dhatu: Fat
- Asthi Dhatu: Bone
- Majja Dhatu: Marrow and nervous tissue
- Shukra Dhatu: Reproductive tissue

Ayurveda explains that our body follows the above chronological order in the process of assimilation or development of our body. It is said Rasa is the first to be formed during the digestion of food. Rasa Dhatu further helps the formation of Rakta Dhatu. Rakta forms the Mamsa and thereafter, Medhas, Asthi, Majja and Shukra are formed in order. It is said that proper formation of the first Dhatu will lead to healthy and vital formation of subsequent Dhatu. Hence it is important that all these metabolic processes are in a healthy order in each of the seven stages.

Stages of Digestion:-
According to Ayurveda digestion is not only happening in the digestive tract but also in the Dhatu or tissues in each part of the body. Ayurveda clearly connects the body.

Prapaka: - This is the first part of food digestion including ingestion, digestion, absorption of food and nutrients.

Vipaka:- This is the second phase of digestion where the nutrients are processed for the formation of Dhatus.

Agni: Agni literally translates as the fire, heat or energy. Ayurveda also explains Agni as an important aspect of digestion. In context to digestion it is known as digestive fire (Pachan-Shakti). Agni is also associated with the biological energy or heat that is governing our output of metabolism, which sustains psycho-physiological life processes. Agni is associated with the digestive enzymes, the metabolic and digestive processes that are taking place as part of breaking down food during the digestion, absorption and assimilation process.

Ayurveda states that "a living being is as old as his 'Agni' or digestive fire. As long as the digestive fire is strong and at its full potential, AMA or toxins cannot be formed and the person remains healthy."

Ayurveda details following Agnis:
1. Jatharagni - Agni associated with ingestion, digestion, absorption and transportation of nutrients in our digestive system.
2. Rasasgni – Agni associated with Plasma and fluids in body.
3. Raktagni – Agni responsible for blood.
4. Mamsagni – Agni associated with muscles and metabolism.
5. Medhagni – Agni governing fat tissue.
6. Ashthigni – Agni responsible for bones and skeletal system.
7. Majjagni – Agni associated with bone marrow and nervous system.
8. Shukragni- Agni responsible for reproductive tissues and fluids.

A healthy and normal digestive process in our body follows the following steps:-
1. Ingestion after proper chewing
2. Breaking down and digestion
3. Absorption of nutrients
4. Excretion of toxic waste.

Due to various physical, mental, emotional stresses and strains, as well as indigestible food, our digestive system cannot follow the proper or full digestion. Ayurveda explains the following causes of unhealthy digestion:

1. Inappropriate food
2. Unhealthy eating habits
3. Weak digestive fire
4. Stresses and strains of life

As our body is not fully digesting food or processing it in a natural manner identified by the intestines or the Dhatus, it leaves the waste or toxic elements in our digestive system and body known as AMA. This half-processed food and toxins in the digestive system, and digestive unmetabolized by-products, circulate in the body as toxins – leading to various health problems (roga-Karana).

Four Types of Agni

Sama-Agni - A Balanced Digestive Fire

- digestion, absorption, and elimination are all at their best and healthy
- Food is easily digested without losing or gaining of weight.
- Feel full of energy and vitality
- Clear, sharp, attentive senses
- Easy elimination of faeces or stool, not too dry or watery.
- Tongue is pink, soft, smooth and moist with little to no white coating in the morning
- No gastric or flatulence issues

Vishama-Agni - Irregular Digestive Fire

- Vata excess digestion
- Fluctuates between lack of hunger or excess of hunger and very random timing
- Erratic behaviour
- Irregular eating patterns and craving for spicy, sweet and salty foods
- May suffer with gas, bloating, gurgling, distention, or constipation
- Underweight or overweight
- Stool tends to be small, dry, or hard
- Brownish-black coating on tongue, which may also be dry, or may have scalloped edges
- Low energy, gets tired easily
- Tends towards feeling ungrounded, fearful, anxious, and insecure

Teekshna-Agni - Sharp Digestive Fire

- Pitta excess type digestion
- Hunger is sharp, fierce, intense and strong
- May suffer with anger and irritation if no food available when hungry
- Hypoglycemic or blood sugar level issues
- May suffer with acid reflux, heartburn, hot flashes, acid indigestion
- Stool is more often soft, loose, may have tendency towards diarrhoea.
- Faeces may be rusty / orange in colour, falls apart, or contains undigested pieces of food in it.
- Yellow coating on tongue with red patches or red spots, or a bright red tongue
- Easily gets tired and often feels hungry
- Judgemental and critical attitude, anger, self-centredness

Manda-Agni - Slow Digestive Fire

- Kapha excess type digestion
- Slow, weak, dull, and sluggish digestion
- Low hunger and easily feels full
- Often skips meals but may eat in excess when bored, depressed or for comfort
- Easily gains weight
- Often suffers with mucous, cough or congestion
- May develop oedema, water retention, nausea, loss of appetite, allergies or obesity
- Stool tends to be soft, dense and heavy, dark brown or black, possibly with mucous
- White coating on tongue, more moisture, excess saliva or slimy coating
- Gets tired and suffers with feeling heavy after eating
- Tends to suffer with depression, attachment, greed, lethargy and dullness of mind

Simple Ayurvedic Recommendations

1. Regular use of some digestive and cleansing herbs like ginger, turmeric, cumin seeds, coriander, mint, Himalayan rock salt, and tulsi in herbal teas or warm drinks.

2. Warm Food and Warm Drinks: Warm water improves our digestive fire. Warm food compared to cold or raw food also improves digestion. Ayurveda uses the term Agni or Fire with digestion and mentions that cold food and drinks extinguish the digestive fire.

3. Prepare and eat your meals with love and gratitude and try to connect with the food.

4. Eat mindfully, chew your food properly and avoid other distractions while eating.

5. We eat to live and grow and hence it should be a sacred practice. Avoid eating on the go if possible and try to make time and sit quietly

with your food, even for a moment, and follow a prayer. At the Ashram we follow the prayer- "aum tat-sat krishnat panamastu", which means "I offer my gratitude to the divine for this nurturing food."

6. Enjoy your meal and try to connect with each of the elements (Pancha-Mahabhutas).

7. Eat heathy, fresh, nutritional and easily digestible food.

8. Cook meals with Ayurvedic herbs like cumin, turmeric, fenugreek, asafoetida, coriander and ajwain seeds.

9. Create a healthy gap between meals and avoid snacking between meals. Ayurveda recommends that we should fast between the meals and not eat anything until the last meal is fully digested.

10 Signs of good food and healthy digestion are feelings of physical lightness, enthusiasm, genuine hunger, a sense of comfort in the body.

11. Avoid comfort eating when you are feeling emotional or distressed.

Swasthya Ke Chatur Stambha (The Four Pillars of a healthy lifestyle) are Ahar (Food), Vihar (Recreation), Achar (Routines), Vichar (Thoughts)

Eka Stambham- Ahaar (First Pillar – Diet)

AHAR means food, diet including drinks. One of the famous Upnishadic statements is "Annam Brahma"—which means the food is Brahman (Divine Source of Creation). There is a famous saying, "We are what we eat and we become what we think". Our food generates the mind and our mind generates the personality. This Swatha Ahara Abhyasa (health food practice) depends on what we eat, how we eat and when we eat. Every bite we put in our mouth counts towards our wellbeing and lifespan quality. Mitahara or eating in moderation is key to maintaining a healthy life.

Ayurveda classifies our food into three categories: Sattvik Ahara, Rajasic Ahara, Tamasic Ahara.

Satvik food is very simple, nutritional, fresh and delicious that gives loads of energy and keeps the body and mind healthy and stable. This food type includes milk and milk products, fresh fruits, dry fruits, seasonal veggies, unrefined cereals, pulses, spices like ginger, pepper, turmeric, cumin, honey, jaggery, ghee and oil

Rajasic food creates a restless state of body and mind. These foods are difficult to digest like non-vegetarian food, non-sprouted beans and pulses, garlic, onion, unseasonal veggies and salt.

Tamasic food gives plenty of energy but also creates a lethargic state of mind. This includes food which is stale or cooked over a long period. This includes refined, processed, artificial flavoured foods, deep-frozen foods, pickles, jams, beverages, deep-fried foods, liquor, tobacco and drugs.

The ancient Hindu scriptures say, "One should break one's night long fast at the time of sunrise and end one's last meal at the time of sunset". Our breakfast should be our first meal and that should be like a king's meal. Whatever we eat in the morning is digested and absorbed to the maximum. Food taken during lunch should be easily digestible and dinner should be the lightest meal of the day.

Our state of mind will decide how food is going to be utilised by the body while we are eating our meal. We should eat our meals with full attention, care and love, chew our food well and enjoy the subtle taste of each food item.

A really important aspect is to avoid any form of distraction while you are eating like using your mobile phone, watching TV or listening to the radio.

Swastha-Dvi-Stambham (The second pillar is Vihar)

Vihar means recreational activities to promote health and joy. Literally Vihara means moving or walking or celebrating. Stress is one of the most common factors as a root cause of many health issues these days. Everybody is stressed on a day-to-day basis. The reasons for stress can vary in each individual and spending time with oneself to de-stress is a big task. Recreation, relaxation and enjoying quality time with family, friends and oneself rejuvenates the body and mind.

Investing some quality time in activities which we enjoy helps clear our mind, relieves stress, depression and anxiety, and elevates our mood giving a feeling of wellbeing. Yoga, meditation, relaxation, music, time in nature, walking, swimming etc. are some quality examples of Vihara.

Active and creative hobbies like gardening, painting, playing musical instruments can help engage all the sensory organs and brain to release old stored unprocessed emotions and recharge the mind. Taking part in sports activities is another way of relaxing the body and mind.

Relaxation and Yoga Nidra is the key to establishing a deep connection with the self and gain a well-balanced personality. Maintain the relaxed attitude throughout the day. Swamiji Dr Gitananda Giri Ji mentions how "relaxation is an art which needs to be cultivated consciously". A regular relaxation practice is important for our body, emotions and our nervous system. Regular exercise and relaxation keeps us fit and helps prevent many health issues.
Swastha-Tri-Stambham- Achara (The Third pillar is Routine)

One of the fundamental principles of success in life involves "Regularity, Repetition, & Rhythm". How often our days can go unplanned, doing nothing or avoiding what we could have done. This leads us to be hassled with too much work or stress at some point. Our mental health and wellbeing are dependent on better and healthy routines (achaar). Regularity and sincerity are two important components of a good routine. We must live like the sun, rising and setting every day without an excuse. We must live like birds and all natural life, doing what they meant to do without an excuse. Following our Dharma.

Learn to organise your life appropriately and follow it sincerely. Whatever you do, do it with full intent, love and care. Incorporate and find balance in all necessary tasks for self, work, food, recreation and sleep.

The solutions to many of our difficulties in life lie in setting out the right habits and right routines. Dr Abdul Kalam has said, "You cannot change your future, but you can change your habits and your habits will surely change your future"

Swastha-Chatur-Stambham (The fourth pillar is Thoughts)
Our mental and intellectual health is dependent on how we think about ourselves, others and the world. Our perceptions, attitudes, belief systems, and values are governing or manifesting factors of life itself. There is plenty of evidence now showing that our biology is dependent upon our psychology.

Our thoughts are food for our mind. Ayurveda mentions that "we are what we eat and we become what we think". If you think you are weak, you will be weak. If you think you are a strong, healthy, happy being you will become healthy, happy and strong. Manage your thought processes appropriately. Reorganise your thoughts, emotions, perceptions and attitude towards yourselves and life. Try to live with an attitude of gratitude and joyfulness.

Positive thoughts, contemplations and affirmations can be added into daily life by reading good books, scriptures, attending Satsangas, reciting mantras, taking part in spiritual ceremonies, recollecting good experiences and thinking positively in all situations.

References and Resources:
1. Yoga Therapy By Dr Ananda Balayogi Bhavanani, www.icyer.com
2. Yoga Step by Step by Swamiji Dr Gitananda Giriji, www.icyer.com
3. Anna Selby; Home Ayurveda Kit; C&B Collins and Brown Publication.
4. Yogacharini Anandhi, Activated Vegan Food, https://activatedveganseminars.com
5. Dr Marc Halpern; Tridosha: The Science Of Ayurveda and the Three Doshas (Vata, Pitta, Kapha); https://www.Ayurvedacollege.com/programs/certification-courses/ayurvedic-health-counselor-1/
6. The Dosha Types in Ayurveda and Reccomendations; https://www.euroved.com/en/Ayurveda/test/vata/#eggs
7. Kristen Schneider, Yoga for Three Doshas; https://www.banyanbotanicals.com/info/blog-the-banyan-insight/details/yoga-for-the-doshas/
8. Charaka Samhita — PV Sharma Translator, Chaukhamba Orientalia, Varanasi, India, 1981, pp. ix-xxxii (I) 4 Volumes

9. Sushruta Samhita — KL Bhishagratna Translator, Chaukhamba Orientalia, Varanasi, India, 1991, pp. iii-lxvi (I), i-xvii (II) 3 Volumes

10. Ashtanga Hridaya — Shri Kanta Murthy Translator, Chaukhamba Orientalia, Varanasi, India, 1991, pp. ix-xxvi 3 Volumes

11. Sharngadhara Samhita — Shri Kanta Murthy Translator, Chaukhamba Orientalia, Varanasi, India, 1984, pp. iii-xvi

12. Madhava Nidanam — Shri Kanta Murthy translator, Chaukhamba Orientalia, Varanasi, India, 1993, pp. iii-xv

13. Bhava Prakasha — Shri Kanta Murthy translator, Chaukhamba Orientalia, Varanasi, India, 1998, pp.vii-xii 2 Volumes

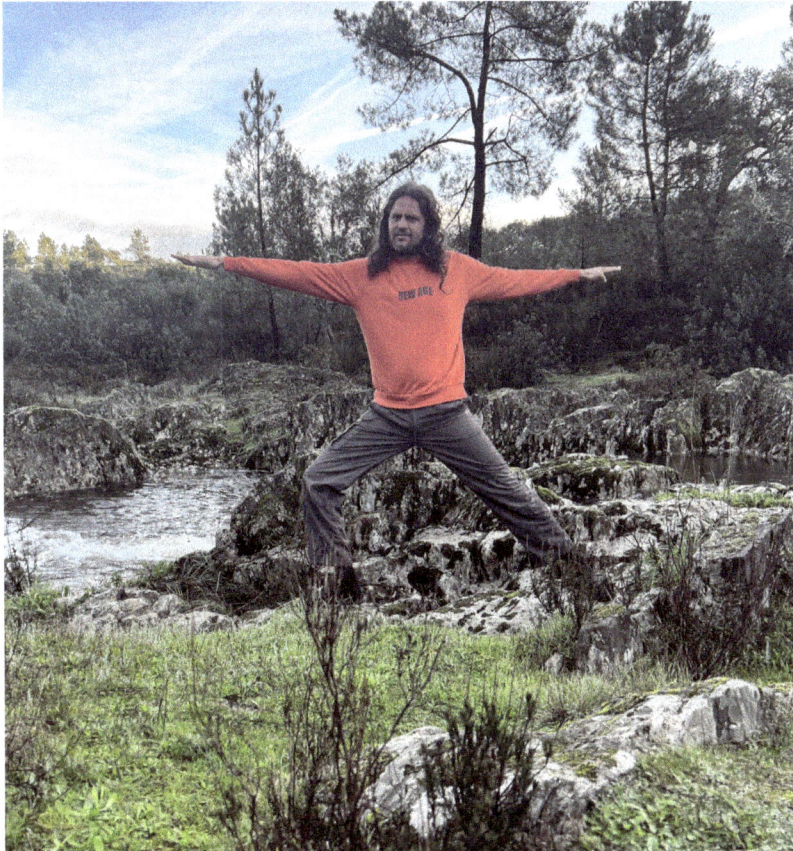

GLOSSARY

Aartava / Aartaya	Egg (female reproductive)
Abhinivesha	Clinging onto life for fear of death
Achar	Healthy activities (such as exercise)
Adhi	Disturbed mind
Adhi-Vyadhi	Psycho-somatic
Agni	Fire or heat
Ahamakara	Ego
Ahar	Healthy, nourishing diet
Ahara	Food, diet or lifestyle
Akasha	Space, ether or voidness
Ama	Toxins
Anahata (Chakra)	Heart Chakra
Anandamaya (Kosha)	Spiritual body, bliss
Angamejayatva	Anxious tremor
Annamaya (Kosha)	Anatomical level of existence
Antaranga (practices)	Inner (yoga), this includes pratyahara, dharana, dhyana and samadhi
Antaraya(s)	Obstacles or hinderances
Antarpushpa	Inner Self
Anuloma-Viloma	Polarity concept in Gitananda Tradition
Anunasika (pranayama)	Nostril cleansing pranayama
Apana vayu	Sub Prana that flows downward toward the lower limbs of the body. Apana vayu is responsible for regulating the outward flow of prana from the body and governs elimination of physical wastes and toxins from the body.
Apunya	Inappropriate actions
Ardha Matsendrasana	Seated twisting postures
Asana(s)	Steady postures
Asmita	False sense of identification
Asthi (Dhatu)	Bones and cartilage, structure
Atman	Self
Avidya	Ignorance
Bahiranga (practices)	External (yoga) practices, this includes yamas, niyamas, asana and pranayama.

Bandhas	Locks for neuromuscular energy
Bhajana	Devotional music or songs
Bhakti Yoga	Devotional service to the divine
Bhastrika (pranayama)	Cleansing breath practice
Bhogi	One who lives life for worldly consumerism
Bhutas	Quality or characteristic
Brahma Danda asana	Seated twisting postures
Buddhi	Intellect
Chakras	Energy centres
Chakrasana	Wheel posture
Chetana	Quality of thought
Chitta Vikshepa	Disturbances in the mind
Daurmanasya	Sadness or dejection
Dhanurasana	Bow pose
Dharana	Concentration, single pointed focus
Dharma	Duty
Dhatus	Tissue (in the body)
Dhyana	Meditation
Dosha	Personal constitution
Drohi	One who is against all of the appropriate life habits
Duhkha	Mental or physical pain, suffering
Garuda Mudra	Eagle arm posture
Guna	Inherent nature or quality
Guru	Teacher or master who guides on the spiritual path
Jala	Liquid or water element
Janusirasana	Seated forward fold over both (outstretched) legs
Jiva	Individual soul
Jnana Yoga	Union through knowledge and wisdom
Jnanendriyas	Five sense organs
Kaivalya	Liberation, enlightenment
Kaki (pranayama)	Crow-peak breath sipping
Kapha	One of the three doshas. Kapha is comprised of earth and water.

Karana Sharira	Casual or karmic body
Karma yoga	Yoga as skilled action performed without expectation
Karmendriyas	Five subtle organs of action (e.g. feet, hands, mouth)
Karuna	Compassion, kindness
Kleshas	Obstacle for growth
Kosha	Layer or sheath
Kriya(s)	Structured movements
Maitri	Friendliness
Majja (Dhatu)	Bone marrow
Mala Shuddhi	Eradication of factors that disturb the balanced working of the body and mind
Malas / Mallas	Waste products
Mamsa / Mansa (Dhatu)	Muscular tissue or flesh
Manda-Agni	Slow digestive fire
Manipura (Chakra)	Solar Plexus Chakra
Manomaya (Kosha)	Psychological level of existence
Medhas (Dhatu)	Fat (in the body)
Meru-Asana	Mountain pose
Mitahara	Moderate eating
Mitahara	Eating in moderation
Moksha	Liberation, enlightenment
Moksha Shastra	Scripture about path of liberation
Mooladhara (Chakra)	Root Chakra
Mudita	Cheerfulness
Mudra(s)	Gestures for energy generation and conservation
Mutra	Urine
Nadi Shuddhi	Purification of all channels of communication
Nadi Sodhana	Deep cleansing pranayama practice
Nadis	Subtle energy channels
Namaskar Mudra	Hands in the prayer position at the heart
Nishkruti	The process of examining the body with the respective Vikriti
Ojas	Spiritual Pranic energy
Pancha	Five

Pancha Kleshas	Psychological afflictions
Pancha Kosha	Five aspects or bodies of our existence
Pancha Mahabhutas	Five elements of the universe (earth, water, fire, air and space)
Pitta	One of the three doshas. Pitta is comprised of fire and water
Posaka	Unstable
Prakriti	Nature, inherent life qualities
Prana	Life force or energy
Pranic	Energy in form of subtlest form of Prana
Prana Vayus	Major energies of physiological function
Pranamaya (Kosha)	Physiological level of existence
Pranayama	Control of energy and breath
Prapaka	First phase of digestion
Prathvi	Earth element
Prathvi Bhuta	Earth element
Prathvi Mudra	Mudra in which the tip of the ring finger and thumb are joined whilst keeping the other three fingers straight.
Pratyahara	Withdrawal of the senses
Prithvi	Earth
Punya	Good deeds
Purisha	Faeces
Purisha Dhara Kala	Membrane that holds the asthi agni
Pwana-Mukta Kriya	Type of kriya to remove deep rooted stress
Raga-Dwesha	Addiction or aversion
Raja Yoga	Yoga of excellence, Royal or highest form of Yoga
Rajas (Guna)	Intense quality, exciting and without limits
Rajasic	Overactive or aggressive
Rakta (Dhatu)	Red blood cells
Rasa (Dhatu)	Plasma and fluid (in the body)
Rogi	One who suffers some form of health issue
Sabija Karma	Seed karma, those who take the seeds and wait for the ideal opportunity to fruit
Sadhakas	Spiritual practitioner

Sama-Agni	Balanced digestive fire
Samadhi	Integrated oneness of yoga
Samadhi Bhavanam	State of integration
Samana	Energy of digestion
Samanya Adhija Vyadhi	Psychosomatic and non-psychosomatic ailments which arise day-to-day
Samatvam	Equanimity
Sankalpa	Aspirations (of the individual)
Sapta Dhatus	Seven substances which make up the body
Sara Adhija Vyadhi	Essential disease of being caught in the birth / congenital disease
Satsangha	Spiritual gathering, lecture
Sattva (Guna)	Ideal, purified quality
Sattvic or Sattwic	Balanced, calm and composed
Savitri Pranayama	Solar rhythmic breath like 6x3x6x3 pattern
Shadrasa	The six flavours
Shanti	Peace
Shat Karmas	Cleansing actions
Shitakari (Pranayama)	Cooling Breath, is a breathing practice that very effectively cools the body, the mind, and the emotions
Shitali (Pranayama)	Cooling Breath, is a breathing practice that very effectively cools the body, the mind, and the emotions
Shukra (Dhatu)	Reproductive tissue
Shvasa Prashvasah	Respiratory irregularities
Sthula Sharira	Gross or physical body
Suka	Pleasure or enjoyment
Sukha Sthanam	Firm and comfortable pose
Sukra	Generative tissue
Sukshma Sharira	Subtle or astral body
Sukshma Sharira	Astral body
Surya Namaskar(s)	Salutations to the sun
Swadhyaya	Self-analysis, self-introspection
Swara	Smooth and regular air flow
Swara Yoga	Yoga of breath and subtle energies

Swatha Ahara Abhyasa	Healthy food practice
Sweda	Perspiration, sweat
Tamas (Guna)	Slow, heavy and dull quality
Tamasic	Dull, lazy or passive
Teekshna-Agni	Sharp digestive fire
Tejas	Male or female hormonal sexual fluids which can be transformed into spiritual energy
Trataka	Concentrated gaze
Tridosha	Three humors
Triguna	The composition of the three Gunas
Trisharira	Threefold aspect of our bodily nature
Tvacha	Skin
Upa Prana Vayus	Minor energies of physiological function
Upasthu	Genitals
Upekshanam	Equanimity
Ustrasana	Camel pose
Vacha	Skin
Vata	One of the three doshas. Vata is comprised of air and space
Vayu	Wind or air element
Veera-Asana	Warrior pose
Veera-Bhadra-Asana	Set of warrior postures
Vichar	Right thoughts and attitude towards life
Vihar	Recreational activities to relax the body and mind
Vijnanamaya (Kosha)	Intellectual level of existence
Vikriti	
Vinyasa	Movement from one asana to another
Vipaka	Second phase of digestion
Vishama-Agna	Irregular digestive fire
Vishuddha (Chakra)	Throat Chakra
Viveka	Rational thinking or discernment
Vriksha-Asana	Tree pose
Vyadhi	Disease
Vyavahar	Healthy relationships

Yama	Niyama
Yoga Chikitsa	Yoga therapy
Yoga Vyayama	Any form of physical, mental or breathing expertise with yogic awareness
Yogi	One who has mastered the mind and remains in inner balance or tranquillity

www.ingramcontent.com/pod-product-compliance
Lightning Source LLC
Chambersburg PA
CBHW071213020426
42333CB00015B/1400